ADRENOMEDULLIN IN CARDIOVASCULAR DISEASE

BASIC SCIENCE FOR THE CARDIOLOGIST

1. B. Swynghedauw (ed.): *Molecular Cardiology for the Cardiologist.* Second Edition. 1998 ISBN 0-7923-8323-0
2. B. Levy, A. Tedgui (eds.): *Biology of the Arterial Wall.* 1999 ISBN 0-7923-8458-X
3. M.R. Sanders, J.B. Kostis (eds.): *Molecular Cardiology in Clinical Practice.* 1999 ISBN 0-7923-8602-7
4. B.Ostadal, F. Kolar (eds.): *Cardiac Ischemia: From Injury to Protection.* 1999 ISBN 0-7923-8642-6
5. H. Schunkert, G.A.J. Riegger (eds.): *Apoptosis in Cardiac Biology.* 1999 ISBN 0-7923-8648-5
6. A. Malliani, (ed.): *Principles of Cardiovascular Neural Regulation in Health and Disease.* 2000 ISBN 0-7923-7775-3
7. P. Benlian: *Genetics of Dyslipidemia.* 2001 ISBN 0-7923-7362-6
8. D. Young: *Role of Potassium in Preventive Cardiovascular Medicine.* 2001 ISBN 0-7923-7376-6
9. E. Carmeliet, J. Vereecke: *Cardiac Cellular Electrophysiology.* 2001 ISBN 0-7923-7544-0
10. C. Holubarsch: *Mechanics and Energetics of the Myocardium.* 2002 ISBN 0-7923-7570-X
11. J.S. Ingwall: *ATP and the Heart.* 2002 ISBN 1-4020-7093-4
12. W.C. De Mello, M.J. Janse: *Heart Cell Coupling and Impuse Propagation in Health and Disease.* 2002 ISBN 1-4020-7182-5
13. P.P.-Dimitrow: *Coronary Flow Reserve – Measurement and Application: Focus on transthoracic Doppler echocardiography.* 2002 ISBN 1-4020-7213-9
14. G.A. Danieli: *Genetics and Genomics for the Cardiologist.* 2002 ISBN 1-4020-7309-7
15. F.A. Schneider, I.R. Siska, J.A. Avram: *Clinical Physiology of the Venous System.* 2003. ISBN 1-4020-7411-5
16. Can Ince: *Physiological Genomics of the Critically Ill Mouse.* 2004 ISBN 1-4020-7641-X
17. Wolfgang Schaper, Jutta Schaper: *Arteriogenesis.* 2004 ISBN 1-4020-8125-1 eISBN 1-4020-8126-X
18. Nico Westerhof, Nikos Stergiopulos, Mark I.M. Noble: *Snapshots of Hemodynamics: An aid for clinical research and graduate education.* 2005 ISBN 0-387-23345-8 eISBN 0-387-23346-6
19. Toshio Nishikimi: *Adrenomedullin in Cardiovascular Disease*, 2005 ISBN 0-387-25404-8 eISBN 0-387-25405-6

ADRENOMEDULLIN IN CARDIOVASCULAR DISEASE

edited by

TOSHIO NISHIKIMI

Department of Hypertension and Cardiorenal Medicine
Dokkyo University School of Medicine
Tochigi, Japan

Springer

Toshio Nishikimi, MD, PhD
Department of Hypertension and Cardiorenal Medicine
Dokkyo University School of Medicine
Mibu, Tochigi
Japan

Library of Congress Cataloging-in-Publication Data

A C.I.P. Catalogue record for this book is available
from the Library of Congress.

ISBN-10: 0-387-25404-8 e-ISBN 0-387-25405-6 Printed on acid-free paper.
ISBN-13: 978-0387-25404-3 e-ISBN 978-0387-25405-0

Printed in the United States of America.

9 8 7 6 5 4 3 2 1 SPIN 11053873

springeronline.com

CONTENTS

Contributing Authors

Ando, Katsuyuki
Department of Nephrology and Endocrinology, University of Tokyo, Tokyo, Japan

Eto, Tanenao
First Department of Internal Medicine, Miyazaki Medical College, University of Miyazaki, Kiyotake, Miyazaki, Japan.

Fujita, Toshiro
Department of Nephrology and Endocrinology, University of Tokyo, Tokyo, Japan

Hirata, Yukio
Department of Clinical and Molecular Endocrinology, Tokyo Medical and Dental University Graduate School, Tokyo, Japan

Horio, Takeshi
Department of Medicine, National Cardiovascular Center, Osaka, Japan

Ishimitsu, Toshihiko
Department of Hypertension and Cardiorenal Medicine, Dokkyo University School of Medicine, Tochigi, Japan

Kangawa, Kenji
Department of Biochemistry, National Cardiovascular Research Institute, Osaka, Japan

Kato, Johji
First Department of Internal Medicine, Miyazaki Medical College, University of Miyazaki, Kiyotake, Miyazaki, Japan.

Kitamura, Kazuo
First Department of Internal Medicine, Miyazaki Medical College, University of Miyazaki, Kiyotake, Miyazaki, Japan.

Matsuoka, Hiroaki
Department of Hypertension and Cardiorenal Medicine, Dokkyo University School of Medicine, Tochigi, Japan

Minami, Junichi
Department of Hypertension and Cardiorenal Medicine, Dokkyo University School of Medicine, Tochigi, Japan

Minamino, Naoto
Department of Pharmacology, National Cardiovascular Research Institute, Osaka, Japan

Nagaya, Noritoshi
Department of Regenerative Medicine and Tissue Engineering, National Cardiovascular Research Institute, Osaka, Japan

Nishikimi, Toshio
Department of Hypertension and Cardiorenal Medicine, Dokkyo University School of Medicine, Tochigi, Japan

Ono, Hidehiko
Department of Hypertension and Cardiorenal Medicine, Dokkyo University School of Medicine, Tochigi, Japan

Shimosawa, Tatsuo
Department of Nephrology and Endocrinology, University of Tokyo, Tokyo, Japan

Shindo, Takayuki
Department of Cardiovascular Medicine, University of Tokyo, Tokyo, Japan

Takahashi, Kazuhiro
Department of Molecular Biology and Applied Physiology,Tohoku University School of Medicine, Sendai, Japan

Tsukada, Kohju
Department of Hypertension and Cardiorenal Medicine, Dokkyo University School of Medicine, Tochigi, Japan

Yoshimoto, Takanobu
Department of Clinical and Molecular Endocrinology, Tokyo Medical and Dental University Graduate School, Tokyo, Japan

Yoshihara, Fumiki
Department of Medicine, National Cardiovascular Center, Osaka, Japan

Introduction

Toshio Nishikimi

The present publication is an up-to-date review of the most relevant aspects of adrenomedullin. It encompasses a broad range of fields, including biochemistry, molecular biology, physiology, pharmacology, pathophysiology of cardiovascular disease, and clinical applications of adrenomedullin to cardiovascular disease. The authors are distinguished colleagues, each one an expert in one or more fields.

The cardiovascular system is regulated by many neurohumoral factors, such as the sympathetic nervous system, renin-angiotensin-aldosterone system, natriuretic peptides, endothelin, and vasopressin. The study of these neurohumoral factors has not only enhanced our understanding of the pathophysiology of cardiovascular disease, but has also contributed to improved diagnosis and therapy. In fact, research on neurohumoral factors led to the development of angiotensin converting enzyme inhibitors, angiotensin receptor blockers, beta-blockers, aldosterone receptor blockers, endothelin antagonists, and recombinant atrial and brain natriuretic peptides, contributing substantially to cardiovascular medicine. Indeed, these drugs are now widely used in daily clinical practice and have become essential for the treatment of patients with cardiovascular disease. Diagnostically, the measurement of atrial and brain natriuretic peptides is a useful tool for evaluating the status of heart failure as well as cardiac remodeling and hypertrophy. Thus, the discovery and evaluation of new hormones has opened new doors leading to further progress in cardiovascular research and medicine.

Adrenomedullin was discovered in 1993 in an extract of human pheochromocytoma while monitoring cAMP levels in rat platelets. Adrenomedullin consists of 52 amino acids and shows slight homology with calcitonin gene-related peptide. More than 1500 peer-reviewed articles have been published regarding its biochemistry, molecular biology, physiology, pharmacology, and pathophysiology over the past 12 years. Because of its actions on the cardiovascular system, adrenomedullin has attracted considerable interest among cardiologists.

Adrenomedullin significantly decreases blood pressure in vivo, directly acts on vascular smooth muscle cells, and increases cAMP levels. Adrenomedullin also acts on vascular endothelial cells and activates endothelial NOS by increasing intracellular Ca^{2+} levels. Thus, adrenomedullin reduces blood pressure indirectly. Strong expression of adrenomedullin mRNA is found in vascular smooth muscle cells and endothelial cells. Its expression in these cells is 20 times higher than that in the adrenal gland. Thus, adrenomedullin is produced and secreted from vascular walls and acts as an autocrine and paracrine factor involved in the regulation of vascular tonus. Furthermore, recent studies suggest a role of adrenomedullin in the pathogenesis of arteriosclerosis.

Not only the vasculature, but also the heart and kidney are considered important target organs of adrenomedullin. Adrenomedullin is expressed in cardiac myocytes, which have abundant adrenomedullin receptors. Indeed, adrenomedullin has positive inotropic action in vivo and in vitro. Adrenomedullin is also expressed in renal tubular cells and glomerular endothelial cells. These cells also have an abundant supply of adrenomedullin receptors. Intrarenal administration of adrenomedullin induces natriuresis, diuresis, and an increase in glomerular filtration rate. Thus, adrenomedullin has a wide variety of unique actions. Recent studies have shown that long-term administration of adrenomedullin or gene delivery of adrenomedullin significantly improves cardiac function, cardiac hypertrophy, and renal disease in hypertension or heart failure. These results suggest that adrenomedullin can be used for the treatment of cardiovascular disease.

The present volume is an effort to summarize our knowledge about adrenomedullin as of the end of 2004. It will hopefully benefit young investigators who specialize in cardiovascular disease and endocrinology.

1

BIOCHEMISTRY OF ADRENOMEDULLIN

Kazuo Kitamura[1], Kenji Kangawa[2], and Tanenao Eto[1]

[1] *First Department of Internal Medicine, Miyazaki Medical College, University of Miyazaki, Kiyotake, Miyazaki, Japan.* [2] *National Cardiovascular Research Institute, Suita, Osaka, Japan*

INTRODUCTION

In 1993, we discovered adrenomedullin (AM) in human pheochromocytoma tissue by monitoring the ability of the cell extracts to increase intracellular cyclic AMP (cAMP) levels in rat platelets. Since then, AM has attracted intense interest from cardiovascular researchers as a result of its multiple biological activities, which include a robust hypotensive effect caused by marked dilation of resistance vessels. AM is biosynthesized and secreted ubiquitously among tissues, including cardiovascular organs, and plasma AM levels are increased in variety of cardiovascular and renal diseases. AM thus appears to function as part of a novel regulatory system that contributes to the control of circulatory and body fluid homeostasis, and may be involved in various pathophysiological changes in cardiovascular diseases. In this chapter, we will focus mainly on the structure of AM, its gene and its distribution, but we will also discuss proadrenomedullin N-terminal 20 peptide (PAMP), another peptide processed from the AM precursor protein.

1. DISCOVERY OF AM

The mammalian cardiovascular system is regulated by subtle mechanisms involving numerous neural and hormonal mediators, including a variety of vasoactive peptides. Consequently, regulation of the cardiovascular function will not be fully understood until all of these vasoactive mediators have been identified and characterized.

With that in mind, we have been searching for peptides that may be relevant to circulatory control using an assay system in which the capacity of substances to elevate cAMP levels in rat platelets was evaluated (Kitamura et al., 1992; Kitamura et al., 1993). Figure 1 shows a cation exchange chromatograph of the low molecular weight fraction of human pheochromocytoma tissue, which contains a group of strongly basic peptides. Four major bioactive peaks and several minor peaks are present. From the major peaks, we were able to isolate vasoactive intestinal peptide (VIP), calcitonin gene related peptide (CGRP) and CGRP-II as endogenous peptides that increase rat platelet cAMP. As all of those peptides are known to be potent vasodilators, we hypothesized that this assay system would useful in a search for as yet unknown vasodilator peptides. And indeed by isolating and sequencing all of the bioactive peaks, we were able to identify AM from a minor peak (Fig. 1). Unfortunately, the amount of peptide thus obtained was so small (20 pmol) that only the N-terminal 18 residues could be determined; everything else about the structure of the peptide remained unknown. In order to obtain a sufficient amount of the peptide for complete analysis, we performed another purification using 40 g of pheochromocytoma tissue, which enabled us to isolate 300 pmol of AM. Because this peptide is also abundant in normal adrenal medulla, it was designated "adrenomedullin" (Kitamura et al., 1993).

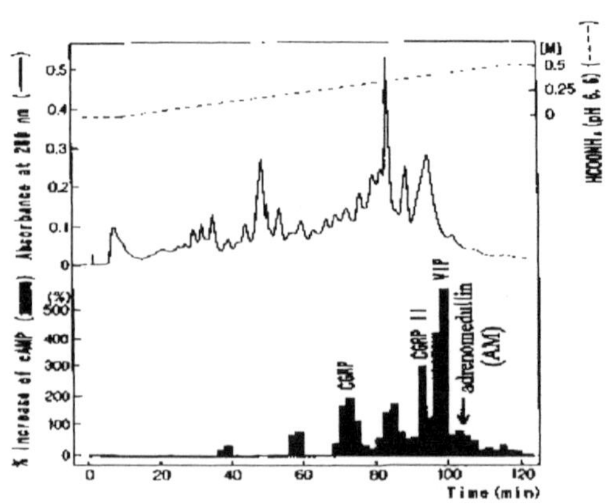

Fig. 1. Discovery of adrenomedullin (AM). Purification of AM from pheochromocytoma extracts. Ion exchange high-performance liquid chromatography of peptides that elevate platelet cAMP. Sample: bioactive fraction from the strong basic peptide fraction (SPIII) from human pheochromocytoma tissue.

2. STRUCTURE OF AM

Human AM is comprised of 52 amino acids and has one intramolecular disulfide bond (Fig. 2) (Kitamura et al., 1993).

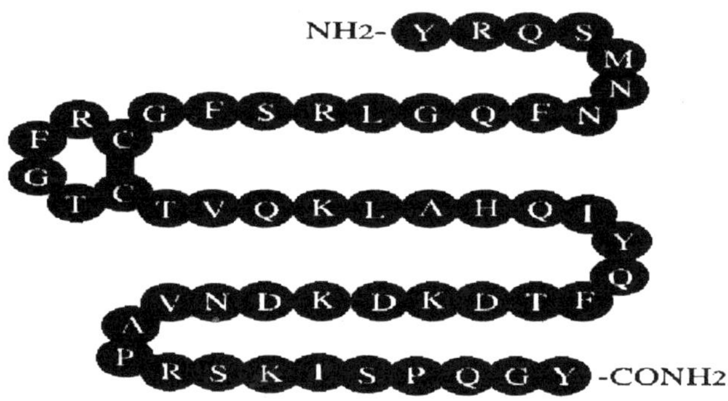

Fig. 2. Structure of human AM.

In addition, the C-terminal Tyr is amidated, which has been observed in a number of other biologically active peptides, including CGRP and amylin, with which AM shares some structural homology. As shown in Fig. 3, the sequence homology of AM with human CGRP (Morris et al., 1984) and amylin (Cooper et al., 1987) is not high, though they share the C-terminal amide and a six residue ring structure formed by the aforementioned intramolecular disulfide linkage. It should be noted that the 14-residue N-terminal extension present in AM is not found in CGRP or amylin. Nevertheless, given the slight sequence homology and pharmacological activities that are similar to those of CGRP, it may be that AM belongs to the CGRP superfamily. Very recently a new member of AM family, adrenomedullin 2 (AM2)/intermedin was identified by two groups (Roh et al., 2004, Takei et al., 2004). Although the sequence identity between AM2/intermedin and AM is rather low (about 30%), the pharmacological activities are similar (Fig. 3).

```
Adrenomedullin      H2N-YRQSMNNFQGLRSFGCRFGTCTVQKLAHQIYQFTDKDKDNV-APRSKISPQGY-CONH2

Adrenomedullin-2/         H2N-TQAQLLRVGCVLGTCQVQNLSHRLWQLMGPAGRQDSAPVDPSSPHSY-CONH2
Intermedin                        *   **  *** ** * *   *          **    **  *

CGRP                              H2N-ACDTATCVTHRLAGLLSRSGGVVKNNF-VPTNVGSKA-F-CONH2
                                       *   **    **          * *   *    *
Amylin                            H2N-KCNTATCATQRLANFLVHSSNNFGAIL-SSTNVGSNT-Y-CONH2
                                       *   **  * **                     *   *
```

Fig. 3. Comparison of amino acid sequence of human AM with human AM 2/intermedin, CGRP and amylin.

In addition to the human peptide, the amino acid sequences of AM from murine, canine, porcine and bovine species have now been determined (Fig. 4).

```
              1        10        20        30        40       50 52
Human     H2N-YRQSMNNFQGLRSFGCRFGTCTVQKLAHQIYQFTDKDKDNVAPRSKISPQGY-CONH2
Porcine   H2N-YRQSMNNFQGLRSFGCRFGTCTVQKLAHQIYQFTDKDKDGVAPRSKISPQGY-CONH2
                                                     *
Dog       H2N-YRQSMNNFQGPRSFGCRFGTCTVQKLAHQIYQFTDKDKDGVAPRSKISPQGY-CONH2
                        *                            *
Bovine    H2N-YRQSLNNFQGLRSFGCRFGTCTVQKLAHQIYHFTDKDKDGSAPRSKISPQGY-CONH2
                  *                          *       **
Rat       H2N-YRQSMN--QGSRSTGCRFGTCTMQKLAHQIYQFTDKDKDGMAPRNKISPQGY-CONH2
                    **  *  *        *                **   *
Mouse     H2N-YRQSMN--QGSRSNGCRFGTCTFQKLAHQIYQLTDKDKDGMAPRNKISPQGY-CONH2
                    **  *  *        *         *      **   *
```

Fig. 4. Comparison of amino acid sequences of AM from several mammalian species.

Porcine AM is nearly identical to the human peptide, with a single substitution (Gly for Asn) at position 40 (Kitamura et al., 1994). Rat AM has 50 amino acids, with 2 deletions and 6 substitutions, as compared with the human peptide (Sakata et al., 1993). Notably, among all these species, the ring structure and C-terminal amide, both of which are essential for biological activity (Eguchi et al., 1994a), are well conserved.

3. STRUCTURE OF AM PRECURSOR

The precursor for human AM (human preproAM) is 185 amino acids in length and includes the AM sequence (Kitamura et al., 1993) (Fig. 5). The predicted sequence of proadrenomedullin (proAM) contains a Gly-Lys-Arg segment immediately adjacent to the C-terminal Tyr residue of AM. GIy-X-Y, where X and Y are basic residues, can serve as a signal for C-terminal amidation, a process in which the glycine residue donates an amide moiety to the free carboxylic acid group in a reaction catalyzed by the enzyme peptidylglycine alpha-amidating monooxygenase (PAM; EC 1.14.17.3) (Bradbury et al., 1991). In addition, the N-terminal region or preproAM contains a unique 20-amino acid sequence that is followed by the amidation signal Gly-Lys-Arg. We deemed it plausible that that a 20-redidue peptide with a C-terminal Arg-$CONH_2$, which we designated "proadrenomedullin N-terminal 20 peptide" (PAMP), could also be processed from the AM precursor. Indeed, we subsequently confirmed that PAMP exists in vivo and exerts a potent hypotensive effect in anesthetized rats.

4. STRUCTURE OF AM GENE

The genes for human and mouse AM have been isolated and their structures determined (Ishimitsu et al., 1994; Okazaki et al., 1996). The AM gene is situated in a single locus on its chromosome. The genomic DNA that includes the human AM gene consists of four exons and three introns (Fig. 5). The mature AM peptide is encoded in the fourth exon, while PAMP is interposed by the second intron. The 5' flanking region of the AM gene contains TATA, CATT and CC boxes, which are regarded as essential to the initiation of transcription by RNA polymerase II and for basal expression of the gene. In addition, there are a number of binding sites for transcriptional regulatory factors, including several for activator protein-2 (AP-2) in the 5' upstream region of exon 1.

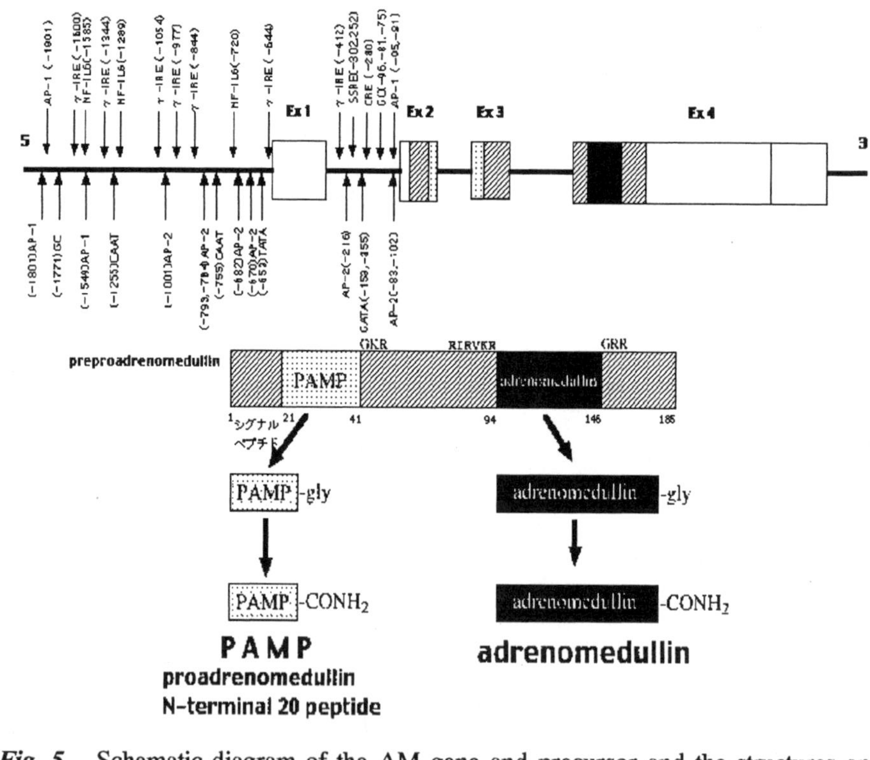

Fig. 5. Schematic diagram of the AM gene and precursor and the structures and biosynthesis of AM and proadrenomedullin N-terminal 20 peptide (PAMP).

That AP-2 mediates transcriptional activation induced by protein kinase C and cAMP suggests that expression of the AM gene is modulated by signal-transduction pathways in which they are components (Imagawa et al., 1987). Given that AM stimulates production cAMP in platelets, the multiple AP-2 sites further suggests the existence of a feedback mechanism affecting AM gene expression. Within intron 1, moreover, there is a consensus sequence for the cAMP-regulated enhancer (CRE) (Fink et al., 1988), which may also be involved in the putative feedback regulation of AM gene expression by cAMP, and nuclear factor-kB (NF-kB) sites have been identified within the AM promoter. In addition, a study of the functional elements of the AM gene revealed that nuclear factor for interleukin-6 (NF-IL-6), AP-2 and the TATA box are all important in the transcriptional regulation of the AM gene (Ishimitsu et al., 1998). Thus, the human AM gene contains components for the regulation of its functional expression, which may be modulated by the activity of protein kinase C and feedback by cAMP.

5. TISSUE DISTRIBUTION OF AM

Although AM was first identified in pheochromocytoma tissue arising from adrenal medulla, immunoreactive AM and AM mRNA has been found to be ubiquitously distributed among various tissues (Fig. 6). Notably, high levels of AM mRNA have been detected in such cardiovascular tissues as atrium, aorta, kidney and lung, though the concentrations of immunoreactive AM in aorta, ventricle and kidney were less than 5% of that seen in adrenal gland (Sakata et al., 1993; Sakata et al., 1994, Sugo et al., 1994). It may be that AM biosynthesized in these tissues is rapidly and constitutively secreted into the blood and/or utilized as an autocrine or paracrine regulator (Bean et al., 1994). By contrast, AM synthesized in adrenal medulla is thought to be stored in the granules and secreted into a regulatory pathway. Thus, the biosynthetic and secretory systems of AM may be tissue-specific.

Immunohistochemical analysis demonstrated the presence of AM immunoreactivity in cardiac myocytes, vascular smooth muscle cells, endothelial cells, renal distal and collecting tubules, mucosal and glandular epithelia of the digestive, respiratory and reproductive systems as well as in the endocrine and neuroendocrine systems

(Martinez et al., 1995; Washimine et al., 1995). In the hypothalamus, AM staining was detected in the supraoptic nuclei and the magnocellular parts of the paraventricular nuclei (Ueta et al., 1995). In addition, immunoreactive AM is present in the blood, urine, cerebrospinal fluid and amniotic fluid (Kitamura et al., 1994; Macri et al., 1996; Nagata et al., 1998).

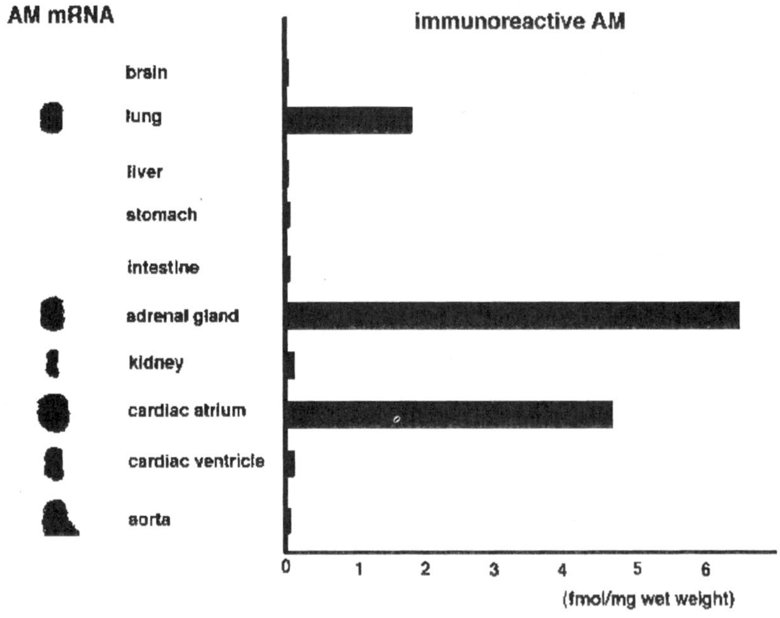

Fig. 6. Distribution of AM mRNA and immunoreactive AM in rat tissue.

6. PRODUCTION OF AM IN CULTURED CELLS

A large number of cultured cell lines produce AM. Reverse transcription-polymerase chain reaction (RT-PCR) analysis revealed the presence of AM in human pulmonary cells, pancreatic islet cells, cardiac myocytes, and vascular endothelial and smooth muscle cells (Sugo et al., 1994; Martinez et al., 1998; Martinez et al., 1995; Tsuruda et al., 1998). Endothelial cells (ECs) actively synthesize and secrete AM (Sugo, 1994), and cultured rat ECs secrete AM at a rate comparable to that of endothelin-1. The presence of specific AM

receptors on vascular smooth muscle cells (VSMCs) (Eguchi et al., 1994) and ECs (Kato et al., 1995) increases our confidence that AM secreted from ECs and VSMCs functions as an autocrine or paracrine regulator mediating vascular cell communication.
Various humoral factors and physical stress appear to stimulate AM synthesis and secretion. Studies in cultured ECs and VSMCs demonstrated that cytokines such as TNF-α and -β, IL-1α and -β, lipopolysaccharide and various circulating hormones, including corticosteroids, thyroid hormones, angiotensin II, norepinephrine, endothelin-1 and bradykinin all strongly stimulate AM production and release (Sugo et al., 1994; Sugo et al., 1995). And shear stress and stretching, acting as a mechanical stimuli, reportedly induce expression of AM mRNA in VSMCs and cardiac myocytes (Chun et al., 1997).

7. PAMP

In its N-terminal region, preproadrenomedullin, the precursor for AM, also contains a unique 20-residue sequence that is followed by the amidation signal Gly-Lys-Arg, which we designated PAMP. Using a radioimmunoassay for the peptide, PAMP was purified from porcine adrenal medulla and human pheochromocytoma, after which the complete amino acid sequence was determined (Kitamura et al., 1994; Kuwasako et al., 1995). In addition to human PAMP, the amino acid sequence of PAMP isoforms from murine, canine, porcine and bovine species have also been sequenced (Fig. 7).

```
Human      ARLDVASEFRKKWNKWALSR-CONH2

Porcine    ARLDVAAEFRKKWNKWALSR-CONH2
                 *
Dog        ARLDVASEFRKKWNKWAVSR-CONH2
                            *
Bovine     ARLDVAAEFRKKWNKWALSR-CONH2
                 *
Rat        ARLDTSSQFRKKWNKWALSR-CONH2
               ** *
Mouse      AGPDTPSQFRKKWNKWALSR-CONH2
            ** ** *
```

Fig. 7. Comparison of the amino acid sequence of proadrenomedullin N-terminal 20 peptide (PAMP) from several mammalian species.

Among these, the amide structure and the amino acid sequence in the C-terminal region, which are required for hypotensive activity, appear to be well conserved. Recently, two major molecular forms of immunoreactive PAMPs were purified from bovine adrenal medulla, and the complete amino acid sequences were determined (Kobayashi et al., 2000). The amino acid sequences of PAMP (1-20) and PAMP (9-20) are identical to these sequences deduced from the cDNA analysis, and the C-terminal Arg were amidated. In humans, the distribution of PAMP is similar to that of AM, most likely due to the fact that both are synthesized from the same precursor (Shimosawa et al., 1997).

PAMP potently and dose-dependently reduces blood pressure in anesthetized rats (Kitamura et al., 1994), and inhibits carbachol-induced catecholamine secretion in cultured bovine adrenal medullary cells (Kobayashi et al., 2000). AM, by contrast, has no effect on catecholamine secretion. Notably, Shimosawa et al. (Shimosawa et al., 1997) demonstrated that AM infused into pithed rat exerts a dose-dependent hypotensive effect, but PAMP does not. Only after the rat's blood pressure was increased to 80-100 mmHg by electrical stimulation did PAMP exhibit a hypotensive effect. Furthermore when peripheral sympathetic nerve activity was enhanced by periarterial electrical stimulation, and noradrenaline released into the perfusate was measured as an indication of neural transmission, PAMP was found to dose-dependently reduce noradrenaline overflow, whereas AM had no effect (Shimosawa et al., 1995). These data suggest that the hypotensive effect of PAMP is likely the result of inhibition of neural transmission rather than via a direct effect on the arteries.

It has been reported that ACTH secretion from cultured rat pituitary cells is inhibited by PAMP (Samson et al., 1998). The effect is dose-related, occurs within a physiologically relevant dose range that is similar to that of AM, and is blocked by the potassium channel blocker, glybenclamide. Both AM and PAMP inhibited evoked aldosterone secretion via direct adrenal actions, though PAMP is significantly more potent than AM (Andreis et al., 1997), and latter also depressed basal aldosterone secretion. CGRP(8-37) abolished the inhibitory action of AM, without affecting that of PAMP.

The receptor for PAMP has never been cloned. However, Iwasaki et al. (Iwasaki et al., 1996) demonstrated PAMP receptors to be widely distributed among rat tissues, and to be most abundant in aorta and adrenal glands. In addition, Ohinata et al. (Ohinata et al., 2000) reported that PAMP showed affinity for gastrin-releasing peptide preferring receptor (GRP-R) and neuromedin B preferring receptor. For instance, PAMP-induced hyperglycemia was inhibited by (D-Phe(6), Leu-NHEt(13), des-Met(14))-BN (6-14), a GRP-R specific antagonist, indicating that the hyperglycemic effect is mediated at least in part via GRP-R. On the other hand, in vivo interaction of PAMP with GRP-R has not yet been detected.

9. CONCLUSION

We have identified a novel hypotensive peptide in extracts of human pheochromocytoma, which we designated "adrenomedullin," as well as another hypotensive peptide, designated "proadrenomedullin N-terminal 20 peptide," which was processed from the same precursor. Although initially isolated from human pheochromocytoma tissue and porcine adrenal medullae, AM has now been detected in a number of organs and tissues, including in the cardiovascular system. Considering the multifunctional characteristics of AM and the fact that plasma immunoreactive AM levels are significantly elevated in patients with cardiovascular disease suggests AM should be recognized as a novel mediator, contributing significantly to the regulation of blood pressure and circulatory homeostasis.

REFERENCES

Andreis, P.G., Mazzocchi, G., Rebuffat, P., Nussdorfer, G.G. (1997) Effects of adrenomedullin and proadrenomedullin N-terminal 20 peptide on rat zona glomerulosa cells. Life Sci., 60: 1693-1697.

Bean, A.J., Zhang, X. and Hoekfelt, T. (1994) Peptide secretion: what do we know? FASEB Journal., 8: 630-638.

Bradbury, A.F., Smyth, D.G. (1991) Modification of the N- and C-termini of bioactive peptides. In: Fricker LD (ed) Peptide Biosynthesis and Processing. CRC Press, Boca Raton, FL,: pp. 231-250.

Chun, T-H., Itoh, H., Ogawa, Y., Tamura, N., Takaya, K., Igaki, T., Yamashita, J., Doi, K., Inoue, M., Masatsugu, K., Korenaga, R., Ando, J., Nakao, K. (1997) Shear stress augments expression of C-type natriuretic peptide and adrenomedullin. Hypertension, 29: 1296-1302.

Cooper, C.J.S., Willis, A.C., Clark, A., Turner, R.C., Sim, R.B. and Reid, K.B.M. (1987) Purification and characterization of a peptide from amyloidrich pancreases of type 2 diabetic patients. Proc. Natl. Acad. Sci. U.S.A., 8: 8628-8632.

Eguchi, S., Hirata, Y., Iwasaki, H., Sato, K., Watanabe, T.X., Inui, T., Nakajima, K., Sakakibara, S., Marumo, F. (1994a) Structure-activity relationship of adrenomedullin, a novel vasodilatory peptide, in cultured rat vascular smooth muscle cells. Endocrinology,135: 2454-2458.

Eguchi, S., Hirata, Y., Kano, H., Sato, K., Watanabe, Y., Watanabe, TX., Nakajima, K., Sakakibara, S., Maruno, F. (1994b) Specific receptors for adrenomedullin in cultured rat vascular smooth muscle cells. FEBS Lett., 340: 226-230.

Fink, J.S., Verhave, M., Kasper, S. Tsukada, T., Mandel, G. and Goodman, R.H. (1988) The CGTCA sequence motif is essential for biological activity of the vasoactive intestinal peptide gene cAMP-regulated Proc. Natl. Acad. Sci. USA., 85: 6662-6666.

Imagawa, M., Chiu, R. and Karin M. (1987) Transcription factor AP-2 mediates induction by two different signal-transduction pathways: protein kinase C and cAMP. Cell, 51: 251-260.

Ishimitsu, T., Kojima, M., Kangawa, K., Hino, J., Matsuoka, H., Kitamura, K., Eto, T. and Matsuo, H. (1994) Genomic structure of human adrenomedullin gene. Biochem. Biophys. Res. Commun., 203: 631-639 .

Ishimitsu, T., Miyata, A., Matsuoka, H., Kangawa, K. (1998) Transcriptional regulation of human adrenomedullin gene in vascular endothelial cells. Biochem. Biophys. Res. Commun., 243: 463-470.

Iwasaki, H., Hirata, Y., Iwashina, M., Sato, K., Marumo, F. (1996) Specific binding sites for proadrenomedullin N-terminal 20 peptide (PAMP) in the rat. Endocrinology., 137: 3045-50.

Kato, J., Kitamura, K., Kangawa, K. and Eto, T. (1995) Receptors for adrenomedullin in human vascular endothelial cells. Eur. J. Pharmacol., 289: 383-385.

Kitamura, K., Kangawa, K., Kawamoto, M., Ichiki, Y. Matsuo, H. and Eto, T. (1992) Isolation and characterization of peptides which act on rat platelets, from a pheochromocytoma. Biochem. Biophys. Res. Commun., 185: 134-141.

Kitamura, K., Kangawa, K., Kawamoto, M., Ichiki, Y., Nakamura, S., Matsuo, H. and Eto, T. (1993) Adrenomedullin: a novel hypotensive peptide isolated from human pheochromocytoma. Biochem.

Biophys. Res. Commun., 192: 553-560.

Kitamura, K., Kangawa, K., Kojima, M., Ichiki, Y., Matsuo, H. and Eto, T. (1994) Complete amino acid sequence of porcine adrenomedullin and cloning of cDNA encoding its precursor. FEBS Letters., 338: 6-10.

Kobayashi, H. Yamamoto, R. Kitamura, K.,Kuwasako, K. Minami, S., Yanagita, T. Shiraishi, S Yokoo, H., Eo, T., Wada, A. (2000) Selective inhibition of nicotinic receptors by proadrenimedullin N-terminal 12 peptide in bovine adrenal chromaffin cells. Molecular brain Reseach, 87: 175-183.

Macri, C.J., Martinez, A., Moody, T.W., Gray, K.D., Miller, M.J., Gallagher, M., Cuttitta, F. (1996) Detection of adrenomedullin, a hypotensive peptide, in amniotic fluid and fetal membranes. Am. J. Obstet. Gynecol., 175: 906-911.

Martinez, A., Cuttitta, F., Teitelman, G. (1998) Expression pattern for adrenomedullin during pancreatic development in the rat reveals a common precursor with other endocrine cell types. Cell Tissue Res., Jul; 293: 95-100.

Martinez, A., Miller, M.J., Unsworth, E.J., Siegfried, J.M., and Cuttitta, F. (1995) Expression of adrenomedullin in normal human lung and in pulmonary tumors. Endocrinology, 136: 4099-4105.

Morris, H.R., Panico, M., Etienne, T., Tippins, J., Girgis, S.I. and Maclntyre, I. (1984) Production of a novel neuropeptide encoded by the calcitonin gene via tissue-specific RNA processing. Nature, 308: 768-748.

Nagata, N., Kato, J., Kitamura, K., Kawamoto, M., Tanaka, N., Eto, T., Takasaki, M. (1998) Dissociation of adrenomedullin concentrations in plasma and cerebrospinal fluid in pregnant and non-pregnant women. Eur J Endocrinol., 139: 611-614.

Ohinata, K., Inui, A., Asakawa, A., Wada, K., Wada, E., Yoshikawa, M. (2000) Proadrenomedullin N-terminal 20 peptide (PAMP) elevates blood glucose levels via bombesin receptor in mice. FEBS Lett., 473: 207-211.

Okazaki, T., Ogawa, Y., Tamura, N., Mori, K., Isse, N., Aoki, T., Rochelle, J.M., Taketo, M.M., Seldin, M.F., Nakao, K. (1996) Genomic organization, expression, and chromosomal mapping of the mouse adrenomedullin gene. Genomics.,: 37: 395-399.

Roh J, Chang CL, Bhalla A, Klein C, Hsu SY. (2004) Intermedin is a calcitonin/calcitonin gene-related peptide family peptide acting through the calcitonin receptor-like receptor/receptor activity-modifying protein receptor complexes. J Biol Chem. 279:7264-7274.

Sakata, J., Shimokubo, T., Kitamura, K., Nakamura, S., Kangawa, K., Matsuo H. and Eto, T. (1993) Molecular cloning and biological activities of rat adrenomedullin, a hypotensive peptide. Biochem. Biophys. Res. Commun., 195: 921-927.

Sakata, J., Shimokubo, T. Kitamura, K., Nishizono, M., Ichiki, Y., Kangawa, K., Matsuo, H., and Eto, T. (1994) Distribution and characterization of immunoreactive adrenomedullin in rat tissue and plasma. FEBS Letters., 352:105-108

Samson, W.K., Murphy, T.C., Resch, Z.T. (1998) Proadrenomedullin N-terminal 20 peptide inhibits adrenocorticotropin secretion from cultured pituitary cells, possibly via activation of a potassium channel. Endocrine., 9: 269-272.

Shimosawa, T., Ando, K., Fujita, T. 1997) A newly identifed peptide, proadrenomedullin N-terminal 20 peptide, induces hypotensive action via pertussis toxin-sensitive mechanisms. Hypertension., 30: 1009-1014.

Shimosawa, T., Ito, Y., Ando, K., Kitamura, K., Kangawa, K. and Fujita, T. (1995) Proadrenomedullin NH2-terminal 20 peptide, a new product of the adrenomedullin gene, inhibits norepinephrine overflow from nerve endings. J. Clin. Invest., 96: 1672-1676.

Sugo, S., Minamino, N., Kangawa, K., Miyamoto, K., Kitamura, K., Sakata, J., Eto, T. and Matsuo, H. (1994a) Endothelial cells actively synthesize and secrete adrenomedullin. Biochem. Biophys. Res. Commun., 202: 1160-1166.

Sugo, S., Minamino, N., Shoji, H., Kangawa, K., Kitamura, K., Eto, T. and Matsuo, H. (1994b) Production and secretion of adrenomedullin from vascular smooth muscle cells. Augmented production by tumor necrosis factor-alpha. Biochem. Biophys. Res. Commun., 203: 719-726.

Takei Y, Inoue K, Ogoshi M, Kawahara T, Bannai H, Miyano S. (2004) Identification of novel adrenomedullin in mammals: a potent cardiovascular and renal regulator. FEBS Lett., 56: 53-58.

Tsuruda, T., Kato, J., Kitamura, K., Kuwasako, K., Imamura, T., Koiwaya, Y., Tsuji, T., Kangawa, K., Eto, T. (1998) Adrenomedullin: a possible autocrine or paracrine inhibitor of hypertrophy of cardiomyocytes. Hypertension, 31: 505-510.

Ueta, Y., Kitamura, K., Isse, T., Shibuya, I., Kabashima, N., Yamamoto, S., Kangawam, K., Matsuo, H., Eto, T., Yamashita, H. (1995) Adrenomedullin-immunoreactive neurons in the paraventricular and supraoptic nuclei of the rat. Neurosci. Lett., 202: 37-40.

Washimine, H., Asada, Y., Kitamura, K., Ichiki, Y., Hara, S., Yamamoto, Y., Kangawa, K., Sumiyoshi, A. and Eto, T. (1995) Immunohistochemical identification of adrenomedullin in human, rat, and porcine tissue. Histochem. Cell Biol., 103: 251-25

2

ADRENOMEDULLIN RECEPTOR AND SIGNAL TRANSDUCTION

Takanobu Yoshimoto and Yukio Hirata

Department of Clinical and Molecular Endocrinology, Tokyo Medical and Dental University Graduate School, Tokyo, Japan

INTRODUCTION

Adrenomedullin (AM) was originally isolated from acid extract of human pheochromocytoma as a bioactive peptide characterized by its ability to raise intracellular cAMP levels in rat platelet (Kitamura et al., 1993). AM shows a partial structural homology with calcitonin gene-related peptide (CGRP) and amylin in terms of the six amino acids ring structure by disulfide bridge and C-terminal amidation, hence AM is classified as a member of calcitonin supergene family (reviewed in Hinson et al., 2000; Poyner et al., 2002). AM was initially characterized as a potent vasodilatory peptide: AM relaxes precontracted vascular bed *in vitro* and intravenous bolus injection of AM caused a potent and long-lasting hypotensive effect *in vivo* (Ishiyama et al., 1993; Kitamura et al., 1993; Nuki et al., 1993; Parkes and May, 1997). However, a growing body of evidence has been accumulated that AM exerts pleiotropic actions, including cell proliferation (Iwasaki et al., 1998a; Shichiri et al., 2003), migration (Fukai et al., 2003; Horio et al., 1995), apoptosis (Kato et al., 1997; Shichiri et al., 1999), inflammation (Hirata et al., 1996; Sugo et al., 1995), angiogenesis (Kim et al., 2003), and hormone secretion (Nussdorfer et al., 1997).

Biological action of AM was initially considered to be mediated solely via cAMP/PKA pathway via its specific receptor, but subsequent studies have revealed that pleiotropic effects of AM are mediated through diverse intracellular signal transduction pathways other than cAMP/PKA pathway, such as ERK/MAPK, PI3K/AKT, and NO/cGMP/PKG pathway. Recently, three novel isoforms of receptor activity-modifying proteins (RAMP) were isolated (McLatchie et al., 1998), and it has been proposed that calcitonin receptor-like receptor (CRLR), a seven-transmembrane receptor, can function as either CGRP receptor or AM receptor, depending on which RAMP isoforms are co-expressed: co-expression of RAMP1 and CRLR confers CGRP1 receptor, whereas RAMP2 or RAMP3 co-expressed with CRLR generates AM receptor (Born et al., 2002; McLatchie et al., 1998; Poyner et al., 2002).

This chapter specifically focuses on the biochemical and molecular characterization of AM receptor, the intracellular signal transduction mechanism of AM in relation to its pleiotropic effects, and current concept of RAMP/CRLR receptor system.

1. CHARACTERIZATION OF AM RECEPTOR

Since biological function of AM was initially characterized as its vasodilator effect *in vitro* and *in vivo*, the receptor of AM was initially studied by its binding to rat VSMCs. By competitive binding assay using [^{125}I] rat (r)AM, we first demonstrated the presence of a single class of binding sites for AM in cultured rat aortic VSMC with the apparent dissociation constant (K_d) of 1.3×10^{-8}M and the maximal binding capacity (B_{max}) of 19,000 sites/cell (Eguchi et al., 1994b). The apparent K_d value is almost comparable concentration to that for AM to induce vasodilation in the perfused rat mesenteric vascular bed (Nuki et al., 1993). Affinity-labeling of VSMC membrane fraction with [^{125}I] rAM revealed two distinct major labeled bands with apparent molecular weight of 120 and 70kDa; both bands disappeared in the presence of excess unlabeled rAM or rat CGRP, suggesting that AM receptor is identical and/or very similar to CGRP receptor (Eguchi et al., 1994b).

Since AM has been shown to increase cAMP generation in rat platelet (Kitamura et al., 1993) and cAMP is a well-known major second messenger for vasodilation, cAMP is originally considered to be a major intracellular signaling molecule for AM. In consistent with this notion, we clearly demonstrated that human (h)AM and rAM dose-dependently (10^{-9}-10^{-6}M) stimulates cAMP formation in rat VSMC with the approximate EC_{50} value (6×10^{-9}M) lower than its K_d value (Eguchi et al., 1994b). CGRP1 receptor antagonist, CGRP(8-37) dose-dependently inhibited cAMP response by rAM and rCGRP (Eguchi et al., 1994b). In agreement with this, AM-induced vasodilator response in rat mesenteric vascular bed was markedly inhibited by CGRP(8-37) (Nuki et al., 1993). Similar inhibitory effect of CGRP(8-37) on AM-induced vasodilation was reported in the isolated rat heart and microvasculature (Entzeroth et al.,1995 ; Hall et al., 1995). AM has been shown to bind with high affinity to, and stimulate cAMP production in neuroblast cell line (SK-N-MC), a cell model exclusively expressing CGRP1 receptor (Zimmermann et al., 1995). These data suggest that at least some biological effect by AM is mediated via CGRP1 receptor. In fact, AM has been shown to compete with [^{125}I]CGRP binding in a variety of tissues, whose affinities are one- or two-orders of magnitude lower than CGRP (Table 1-A and 1-B), suggesting the preferential binding of AM to CGRP1 receptor.

In contrast, using [^{125}I] AM binding studies, the presence of specific AM binding sites with much higher affinity to AM than CGRP, has been reported (Table 1). For example, [^{125}I] rAM binding to rat lung and heart membranes was competed by rAM with high affinity (Ki: 5.8 and 0.2nM, respectively), whereas rCGRP could not or scarcely compete with [^{125}I] rAM binding to these tissues (Owji et al., 1995). It is of note, however, that rAM competed with [^{125}I]CGRP binding to the same tissue preparations with relatively high affinity (Owji et al., 1995). These data clearly demonstrated the presence of specific AM receptors in lung and heart, in addition to the specific CGRP receptors with relative high-affinity to AM. Similar results were also noted in L6 cells and spinal cord (Coppock et al., 1996; Owji et al., 1996). [^{125}I]AM binding studies obviously revealed that CGRP was about three orders of magnitude less than AM, suggesting highly specific receptors for AM. Since a wide variety of cells and tissues, including lung, heart, and vascular tissue, have both specific CGRP and AM binding sites, it is difficult to distinguish between two distinct, but very similar receptors in these tissues. Collectively, AM appears to exert its biological effect through its specific AM receptor and/or CGRP1 receptor.

Table 1-A and 1-B Characterization of AM and CGRP binding site

1-A. [^{125}I]CGRP binding site

Tissue or cell	CGRP affinity (nM)	AM affinity (nM)	Ref
Rat lung	0.3 (IC_{50})	5.0 (IC_{50})	Owji et al., 1995
Rat heart	0.05 (IC_{50})	0.8 (IC_{50})	Owji et al., 1995
SK-N-MC cells	0.04 (Ki)	0.37(Ki)	Entzeroth et al., 1995
	3.5 (Ki for CGRP(8-37))		
L6 cells	0.13 (IC_{50})	8.7 (IC_{50})	Coppock et al., 1996
Rat spinal cord	0.18 (Kd)	34.6 (Ki)	Owji et al., 1996
Rat uterus	0.14 (Kd)	1.67 (Ki)	Upton et al., 1997
Rat hypothalamus	0.1 (Kd)	4.6 (Ki)	Taylor et al., 1996
	4.0 (Ki for CGRP(8-37))		

1-B. [^{125}I]AM binding site

Tissue or cell	AM affinity(nM)	CGRP affinity(nM)	Ref
Bovine aortic EC	10*	>1000	Shimekake et al., 1995
Rat lung	1.3 (IC_{50})	>1000	Owji et al., 1995
Rat heart	0.5 (IC_{50})	1050	Owji et al., 1995
Swiss 3T3 cell	3.5 (IC_{50}	>1000	Withers et al., 1996
Rat aorta	1.38 (Kd)	>1000	Nandha et al., 1996
Rabbit kidney	0.45 (IC_{50})	>1000	Hjelmqvist et al., 1997
Rat-2 fibroblast	0.43 (Kd)	>1000	Coppock et al., 1999
Human brain	0.17 (Kd)	>1000	Sone et al., 1997
L6 cells	0.22 (IC_{50})	>1000	Coppeck et al., 1996
Rat uterus	0.08 (Kd)	>1000	Upton et al., 1997

IC_{50}: concentration inhibiting binding by 50%; Ki: absolute inhibition constant; Kd: dissociation constant; *exact IC_{50} could not be calculated.

2. STRUCTURE-ACTIVITY RELATIONSHIP OF AM

Although the structural homology between AM and CGRP is low (~30%), calcitonin supergene family share the ring structure formed by an intramolecular disulfide bond and amidated C-terminal Tyr^{52} residue in common (reviewed in Hinson et al., 2000; Poyner et al., 2002). Hence, we studied structure/activity relationship of AM molecule using various synthetic human AM analogs in rat VSMCs (Table 2) (Eguchi et al., 1994a). Comparison between binding affinities and potencies of adenylate cyclase activity by synthetic AM analogs are summarized in Table 2. N-terminal-truncated derivatives, hAM-(13-52)-NH_2 and hAM-(16-52)-NH_2, both retaining the cyclic structure and the amidated C-terminus showed comparable Ki and cAMP-generating activities to those of mature form hAM-(1-52)-NH_2, whereas N-terminal fragment hAM-(1-10)-OH had no effect. These data indicate that N-terminal residues (1-15) of AM molecule are not essential for interaction with its receptor. Both removal of the C-terminal Tyr^{52} residue [hAM-(1-51)-OH] and [hAM-(1-52)-OH] resulted in a remarkable decrease in receptor-binding activity and cAMP response. The amidation of the C-terminal Gly^{51} residue [hAM-(1-51)-NH_2] retained some, although less potent than hAM-(1-52)-NH_2, receptor-binding activity and cAMP response, indicating the importance of C-terminal amidation rather than the amidated Tyr^{52} residue *per se*. Cleavage of the disulfide bond between the Cys^{16} and Cys^{21} residue by carbamoylmethylation [[Cys(CAM)^{16,21}]hAM-NH_2] retained some, although less potent than hAM-(1-52)-NH_2, receptor-binding activity, but completely lost cAMP response. Collectively, our data indicates that amidation of C-terminal residue and the cyclic structure of AM molecule are critical for receptor binding and cAMP response.

Table 2 Comparison between binding affinities and potencies of adenylate cyclase activity by hAM analogs

hAM analogs	Ki(_M)[a]	EC_{50}(_M)[b]
hAM-(1-52)-NH_2	0.023	0.03
hAM-(13-52)-NH_2	0.039	0.03
hAM-(16-52)-v	0.062	0.03
hAM-(1-51)-NH_2	0.27	0.24
hAM-(1-52)-OH	1.0	>1.0
hAM-(1-51)-OH	1.1	>1.0
Cys(CAM)^{16,21}]hAM-NH_2	1.3	>1.0
hAM-(22-52)- NH_2	1.6	>1.0
hAM-(33-52)- NH_2	>1.0	>1.0
hAM-(1-10)-OH	>1.0	>1.0
hAM-(1-10)-OH	>1.0	>1.0

[a]The apparent inhibition constant (Ki) obtained from [^{125}I] hAM binding studies.

[b]The appropriate half-maximal effective concentration (EC50) obtained from adenylate cyclase stimulation. Reproduced with permission from ref. (Eguchi et al., 1994a).

CGRP(8-37), which lacks N-terminal ring structure but retains C-terminal portion of CGRP, has been widely recognized and used as a CGRP1 receptor antagonist. In the same analogy, we designed hAM-(22-52)-NH_2, which lacks N-terminal ring structure but retains C-terminal portion. We found that hAM-(22-52)-NH_2 retain receptor binding activity, but devoid of cAMP response (Eguchi et al., 1994a). In addition, hAM-(22-52)-NH_2 inhibited hAM-stimulated cAMP formation with apparent IC_{50} ($4x10^{-6}$M). Hence, we proposed that hAM-(22-52)-NH_2 serves as a selective antagonist for AM receptor.

3. DISCOVERY OF CRLR/RAMP SYSTEM

In 1991, calcitonin (CT) receptor was identified as the first CT supergene family receptor by the expression cloning system from the cDNA library of a porcine kidney epithelial cell line (Lin et al., 1991). CT receptor belongs to type B (Class II) family of G protein coupled receptor (GPCR), including PTH, glucagon, and CRF receptors. These receptors are characterized by the long extracellular N-terminal domain containing several cysteine, the intracellular carboxy-terminal domain lacking the palmitoylation site, and capability of cAMP generation through activation of Gs (Gether, 2000).
Shortly after the molecular cloning of CT receptor, calcitonin receptor-like receptor (CRLR) was identified by PCR cloning from rat hypothalamus by utilizing the homology between type B family Gapers (Njuki et al., 1993). Subsequently, human and other mammalian CRLR homologues were also cloned (Aiyar et al., 1996; Elshourbagy et al., 1998; Fluhmann et al., 1995), which exhibit 50~60% sequence homology with the CT receptor of the same species. In initial transfection studies using several mammalian cells, CRLR showed no affinity to any member of known CT supergene family (Fluhmann et al., 1995; Njuki et al., 1993), thus initially considered as an orphan GPCR. However, Aiyar et al. have shown that human CRLR exhibits the pharmacology of CGRP1 receptor when stably transfected into the cell line derived from human embryonic kidney cell line, HEK293 (Aiyar et al., 1996). This finding was further confirmed using rat and porcine CRLR in transfected HEK293 (Elshourbagy et al., 1998; Han et al., 1997), suggesting that HEK293 cells could express certain endogenous factor(s) essential for the functional expression of CRLR.

This assumption was then confirmed by the discovery of a novel transmembrane protein, termed receptor activity modifying protein (RAMP) (McLatchie et al., 1998). The introduction of cRNA from SK-N-MC cells, where CGRP1 receptor is abundantly present, into Xenopus oocyte induced the novel cAMP response to CGRP. The identified cDNA encoded the 148 amino-acid residues with a single transmembrane domain, named RAMP1. Subsequent study showed that co-transfection of CRLR and RAMP1 into COS-7 cells exhibits functional CGRP1 receptor, whereas the transfection of either gene alone shows no effect (McLatchie et al., 1998). In addition, two additional members of RAMP family were also identified through database search, named RAMP2 and RAMP3 (McLatchie et al., 1998). Although sequence similarity between three RAMP isoforms are less than 30% within the same species, all three isoforms share the conserved cysteine residues at their extracellular domain and DPPXX and LVVWXSK sequences flanking the transmembrane domain, whose functional role remains unknown (Born et al., 2002).

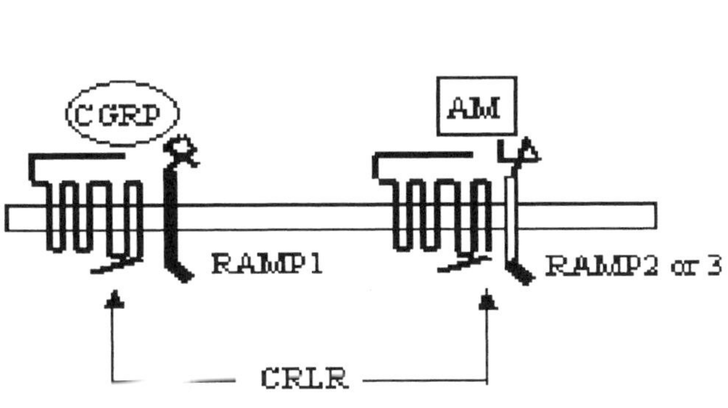

Fig. 1 CRLR and RAMP isoform determine the ligand selectivity for CGRP and AM. Extracellular domain of RAMPs plays an important role in ligand selectivity. Glycosylation of CRLR is important for its cell surface localization, but not for its ligand selectivity.

Co-transfection of CRLR and RAMP2 or RAMP3 exhibits functional AM receptor with high affinity to AM, but not to CGRP. RAMP2 and RAMP3 appears to be indistinguishable from each other in terms of AM binding and cAMP response (McLatchie et al., 1998). Collectively, co-expression of

CRLR with RAMP1 and RAMP2/3 exhibits the CGRP1 receptor and AM receptor pharmacology, respectively (Fig. 1).

4. CRLR/RAMP INTERACTION: RECEPTOR MODIFICATION AND THE MECHANISM OF LIGAND SPECIFICITY

McLatchie et al. initially showed that RAMPs are required to transport CRLR to the plasma membrane (McLatchie et al., 1998). Co-expression of CRLR and RAMP1 exhibited mature glycosylated receptor with CGRP1 receptor property, whereas co-expression of CRLR and RAMP2 or 3 resulted in core-glycosylated receptor with AM receptor property. Hence, the ligand specificity of the receptor formed by CRLR/RAMPs has been initially thought to be determined by the glycosylation pattern of the receptor (McLatchie et al., 1998). However, in Drosophila Schneider (S2) cells stably co-transfected with CRLR and RAMP1 or 2 revealed the pharmacology of CGRP1 receptor and AM receptor, respectively, although both receptors were uniformly glycosylated independent of RAMP1 and 2 expression (Aldecoa et al., 2000). The subsequent study confirmed that RAMP2 and 3 also facilitate full maturation and terminal glycosylatin of CRLR, and only the fully-processed receptor is capable of interacting with AM and CGRP. In other words, although co-expression of CRLR and RAMP2 resulted in increase in core-glycosylated CRLR at whole cell levels, only the fully-processed CRLR could express on cell surface (Hilairet et al., 2001). Thus, it is currently recognized that the glycosylation pattern itself does not appear to determine the ligand selectivity of CRLR/RAMP system as initially speculated, but the glycosylation of CRLR is essential for the cell surface localization of CRLR (Flahaut et al., 2002). By contrast, the CRLR-RAMP heterodimer assembly is indispensable for the cell surface localization of RAMP1 (Christopoulos et al., 1999; Flahaut et al., 2002).
The co-transfection of CT receptor and RAMP1 or 3 was shown to exhibit the pharmacology of amylin receptor, suggesting that RAMP is involved in the determination of the functional property of Class II GPCR (Christopoulos et al., 1999; Muff et al., 1999). The ligand-receptor crosslinking study revealed RAMP-ligand complex as well as CRLR-ligand complex, suggesting that not only CRLR but also RAMP comprises the ligand recognition site of the receptor with the formation of ligand-CRLR-RAMP complex. The study using confocal microscopy also revealed the

ligand-CRLR-RAMP co-localization on the cell surface (Leuthauser et al., 2000). Recent work using RAMP1 extracellular domain as a chimera with PDGF receptor transmembrane domain clearly reveals that extracellular domain of RAMP is sufficient for assembling functional CGRP receptor (Fitzsimmons TJ et al., 2003). It has been very recently revealed that transfection of deletion mutants (residues 91-94, 96-100, or 101-103) of hRAMP1 blocked CGRP binding and cAMP response, whereas substituting aranine for the residues 91-103 one at a time had little effects on CGRP response (Kuwasako et al., 2003). It is therefore suggested that structural conformation of RAMP or its allosteric effect on CRLR rather than individual amino acid sequence play a pivotal role in the determination of ligand specificity.

It has been also shown that CRLR interacts with another protein, receptor component protein (RCP), identified as the protein which confers the CGRP-mediated cAMP response in *Xenopous laevis* oocyte, in a similar manner as does RAMP1 (Luebke et al., 1996). There is no sequence similarity between RCP and RAMPs. It is thus intriguing that RCP could interacts with CRLR and anti-sense oligonucleotides for RCP decreased the CGRP response in NIH3T3 cell line (Prado et al., 2001; Evans et al., 2000). Furthermore, RAMP/CRLR/RCP complex formation was confirmed by immunoprecipitation experiment (Prado et al., 2001). These data suggest that RCP may play a pivotal role in AM/CGRP receptor system, however, further study is required to establish its biological significance.

5. cAMP/PROTEIN KINASE A (PKA) PATHWAY

(1) VASODILATION

Since the discovery of AM (Kitamura et al., 1993), cAMP was initially considered to be a major intracellular signaling molecule for AM. We have first demonstrated that AM activates adenylate cyclase in rat VSMC (Eguchi et al., 1994a; Eguchi et al., 1994b); cAMP response by AM was enhanced by exogenous addition of GTP, and AM receptor binding was inhibited by a non-hydorlyzable GTP analog, GTP-gS (Eguchi et al., 1994a). Furthermore, the cAMP response by AM was shown to be abrogated by pretreatment with cholera toxin, but not by pertuissis toxin, suggesting that

AM receptors are functionally coupled to adenylate cyclase via the stimulatory G-protein (Gs) (Eguchi et al., 1994a). Our data from the pharmacological experiments have been confirmed by the molecular identification of AM receptor, CRLR-RAMP system (Born et al., 2002; Poyner et al., 2002), where CRLR belongs to family B of GPCR as characterized by functional coupling to Gs (Gether, 2000). Co-expression of CRLR and RAMP1 exhibits the cAMP response by CGRP, whereas RAMP2 or 3 co-expressed with CRLR exhibits cAMP response specifically by AM (McLatchie et al., 1998).

(2) MITOGENIC ACTION

AM exerts its mitogenic action via cAMP/PKA pathway in Swiss 3T3 cells; AM increase DNA synthesis and cell proliferation, whose effect was abolished by a PKA inhibitor (H-89) (Withers et al., 1996). Furthermore, transfection of constitutive active mutant of Gs_ mimicked the mitogenic response by AM (Withers et al., 1996). Similar mitogenic response by AM through cAMP/PKA pathway has been shown in human oral keratinocyte (Kapas et al., 1997). On the other hand, cAMP/PKA pathway is widely recognized as a negative regulator of cell growth. In accordance with this, it has been shown that AM inhibits DNA synthesis via cAMP-dependent pathway in serum stimulated growing VSMCs (Kano et al., 1996). A similar anti-mitogenic action by AM has been reported in cultured mesangial cells (Chini et al., 1995; Segawa et al., ; Togawa et al., 1997), whose effect was mediated via cAMP/PKA pathway. We also confirmed that AM caused a partial inhibition of cell growth when AM is added to asynchronously growing VSMC supplemented with serum containing several growth factors (Iwasaki et al., 1998a; Shichiri et al., 2003). Collectively, it is suggested that bi-functional role of AM for cell growth control; in quiescent cells AM exerts its mitogenic action via PTK/ERK pathway (as discussed in the following section), whereas AM exerts its anti-mitogenic action via cAMP/PKA pathway in asynchronously growing cells (Fig. 2). Thus, AM appears to play dual roles in cell growth, depending on the cell type and cell cycle stage.

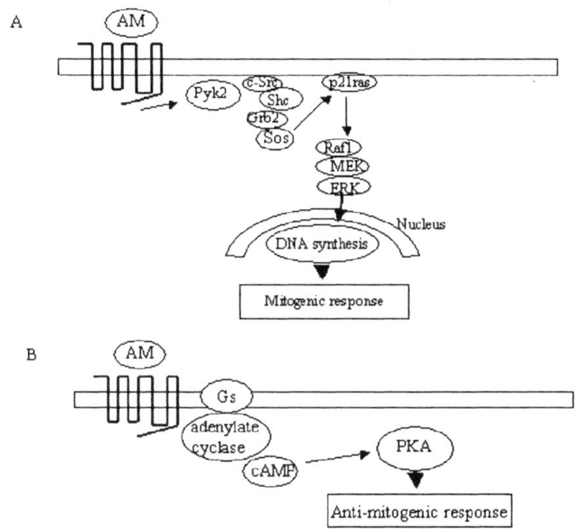

Fig. 2 Dual effect of AM on cell proliferation in VSMC. A: AM activate Pyk2/c-src non-receptor tyrosine kinase pathway, leading to activation of Ras/MEK/ERK pathway and cell proliferation. B: AM stimulate cAMP-PKA pathway, leading to growth inhibition in cells, in which ERK activation pathway is not linked to AM response.

(3) ANTI-OXIDANT ACTION

It has recently been shown that administration of salt and angiotensin II (Ang II) to AM deficient mice generated by gene targeting resulted in perivascular inflammation in coronary artery and increases in systemic and local oxidative stress and reversal of increased urinary isoprostane excretion, an oxidative stress marker, by exogenous AM supplementation (Shimosawa et al., 2002). These data postulate the notion that AM may play a protective role against oxidative stress as an endogenous anti-oxidant *in vivo*. However, the underlying cellular mechanism and the mode of action by AM have not been clarified yet. Therefore, we have explored the underlying molecular mechanism of the putative anti-oxidant action of AM against Ang II-induced reactive oxygen species (ROS) generation in rat VSMCs

(Yoshimoto et al., 2004). Using DCF fluorescence that detects ROS, AM inhibited intracellular ROS generation by Ang II, , whose effect was mimicked by dibutyl cAMP and inhibited by PKA inhibitor (H-89) and a receptor antagonist, CGRP(8-37). Thus, our data demonstrate that AM directly inhibits intracellular ROS generation via AM receptor-mediated and cAMP/PKA pathway in VSMC, suggesting its protective role as an endogenous anti-oxidant in Ang II-induced vascular injury (Fig. 3).

As for the regulation of vascular AM receptor, we have demonstrated distinct desensitization of adenylate cyclase coupled to AM receptor (Iwasaki et al., 1998b). The cAMP response by AM was markedly decreased by pretreatment with AM in a dose-dependent manner. Receptor desensitization occurs in a variety of GPCRs (Wang et al., 1990). For example, phosphorylation of beta–adrenoceptor by PKA and by a GPCR kinase mediates heterologous and homologous desensitization of the adenylate cyclase in response to beta–adrenergic agonist, respectively (Benovic et al., 1985; Hausdorff et al., 1989). However, the homologous desensitization of vascular AM receptor was independent of PKA, protein kinase C (PKC), protein tyrosine kinase (PTK) or receptor sequestration, since pretreatment with each of these inhibitors failed to affect the AM-stimulated cAMP response (Iwasaki et al., 1998b). Thus, the mechanism(s) responsible for the homologous desensitization of vascular AM receptor remains to be determined.

Intracellular cAMP generation by AM and other CT supergene family has been recognized as a major signal transduction for their biological effects. However, a growing body of evidence has been accumulated and showing that cAMP/PKA pathway does not necessarily account for all of the biological actions by AM. Although cardiovascular effects by AM, such as vasodilation, and positive inotropic action, are usually accompanied by increased cAMP response, there have been only a few studies showing that such AM's actions could be blocked by either cAMP antagonists or PKA inhibitors. Furthermore, we have shown that AM has pleiotropic effects other than cardiovascular effects, such as cell growth (Iwasaki et al., 1998a; Shichiri et al., 2003), migration (Fukai et al., 2003), and apoptosis (Kato et al., 1997; Shichiri et al., 1999), whose effects are independent of cAMP/PKA pathway. Thus cAMP/PKA pathway accounts for many, but not all, biological actions by AM, however, the importance of signal transduction pathways other than cAMP/PKA pathway needs to be taken into much consideration.

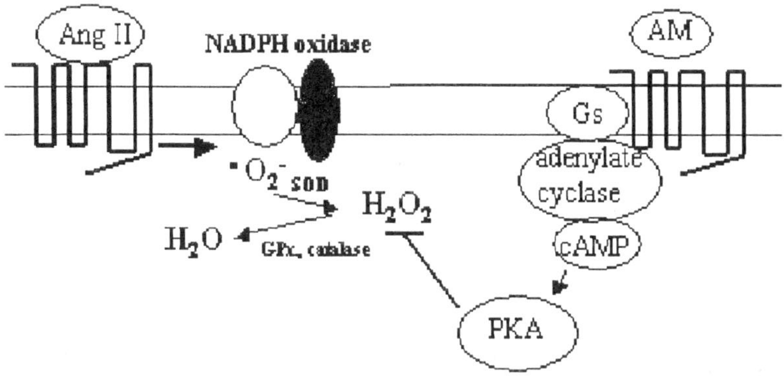

Fig. 3 Anti-oxidant effect of AM. In VSMC AM directly inhibits intracellular ROS generation by Ang II via its receptor-mediated and cAMP/PKA dependent mechanism.

6. PROTEIN TYROSINE KINASE (PTK)/ EXTRACELLULAR RGULATED KINASE (ERK) PATHWAY

The mitogenic effect of AM has been demonstrated in a variety of cells, including certain tumor cell lines, VSMC, fibroblasts, keratinocytes, osteoblasts, adrenal zona glomerulosa cells and so forth. The possible role of AM as an autocrine/paracrine growth factor has been suggested for various tumor cell lines (Martinez et al., 1997; Miller et al., 1996; Takahashi et al., 1997a; Takahashi et al., 1997b). We demonstrated for the first time that AM stimulated DNA synthesis and cell proliferation in quiescent rat VSMC, whose effect was inhibited by CGRP(8-37) (Iwasaki et al., 1998a; Shichiri et al., 2003). Furthermore, AM rapidly and transiently stimulated ERK activities; the AM-induced mitogenic effect and ERK activation was completely blocked by a MEK inhibitor (PD98059) and a protein tyrosine kinase (PTK) inhibitor (genestein). Our data strongly suggest that the mitogenic effect of AM on VSMCs is mediated via PTK/ERK pathway. It is of note that a cAMP antagonist (Rp-cAMP-S) and a highly selective PKA inhibitor (KT5720) failed to inhibit the mitogenic effect and ERK activation by AM, despite of the AM-mediated cAMP response. In our study, AM had no effect on either intracellular Ca^{2+} concentration ($[Ca^{2+}]i$) or inositol 1,4,5,-

triphosphate formation, and a selective PKC inhibitor (GF109203X) and a dihydropyridine-sensitive Ca^{2+} channel blocker (nicardipine) failed to block AM-induced ERK activation. Collectively, our data suggest that AM exerts its mitogenic activity via PTK-mediated ERK activation in quiescent VSMC (Iwasaki et al., 1998a).

Our results with PTK-dependent ERK activation by AM independent of Ca^{2+} and PKC, suggests that AM activates receptor and/or non-receptor PTK cascade, thereby leading to Ras-dependent MEKK-MEK-ERK pathway. In consistent with this notion, AM rapidly induced tyrosine phosphorylation of several proteins (120kDa, 90kDa, 50kDa) (Iwasaki et al., 1998a). Subsequently, we identified the 120kDa tyrosine-phosphorylated protein as proline-rich protein kinase 2 (Pyk 2), a non-receptor PTK (Iwasaki et al., 2001). AM rapidly (within 1 min) phosphorylates Pyk 2, followed by a gradual decline to the basal level by 10 min; the time course of Pyk 2 phophorylation was identical with its kinase activity as confirmed by immuno-complex kinase assay. Furthermore, immunoprecipitation studies revealed that Pyk 2 activation induced interaction with and activation of c-Src, a non-receptor PTK, subsequently leading to complex formation with adaptor proteins (Shc and Grb2). These adaptor protein complex recruits SOS, a GTP exchange protein for Ras, finally leading to sequential activation of Ras-MEKK-MEK-ERK cascade (Iwasaki et al., 2001). Our data demonstrated for the first time the involvement of non-receptor PTK/ERK pathway in VSMCs in the mitogenic action by AM (Fig. 2). A growing body of evidence thus far accumulated has revealed that AM is a potent mitogen for activity on various tumor and non-tumor cells (Hinson et al., 2000; Shichiri and Hirata, 2003).

7. NO/cGMP/PROTEIN KINASE G (PKG) PATHWAY

Several lines of evidence have been accumulated showing that vasodilator action of AM is mainly mediated via endothelial nitric oxide (NO) production, because vasodilatory effects by AM in several vasculatures are blocked by NO synthase (NOS) inhibitors (Hinson et al., 2000; Kitamura et al., 2002). In bovine endothelial cells, AM was shown to activate phospholipase C via Gq protein to increase $[Ca^{2+}]_i$, possibly leading to activation of Ca^{2+}-depndent endothelial NOS (Shimekake et al., 1995). Since NO activates soluble guanylate cyclase to increase intracellular cGMP levels in VSMC, cGMP-dependent protein kinase (PKG) could function as a major signaling molecule for AM-induced vasorelaxation.

8. PI3 KINASE/AKT PATHWAY

A recent study has shown that AM exerts NO-dependent vasodilation through PI3 kinase/AKT pathway (Nishimatsu et al., 2001). Furthermore, several studies have shown that AM plays a protective role in ischemia-reperfusion myocardial injury via PI3 kinase/AKT pathway (Okumura et al., 2004; Yin et al., 2004). We also observed that mitogenic response of AM in VSMCs is blocked by PI3 kinase inhibitors (wortmannin, LY294002) in the same manner as MEK inhibitor (Shichiri et al., 2003). These data are consistent with the notion that PI3 kinase/AKT pathway plays a pivotal role in certain biological actions by AM, although further studies are required to elucidate how the PI3 kinase is activated following AM stimulation.

9. UNKNOWN SIGNAL TRANSDUCTION PATHWAY(S) FOR APOPTOSIS AND MIGRATION

(1) ANTI-APOPTOTIC EFFECT

After serum-deprivation, endothelial cells undergo apoptosis. We demonstrated for the first time that AM acts as an anti-apoptotic factor for rat aortic endothelial cells (RAECs) in a dose-dependent manner (Kato et al., 1997), although it has no mitogenic effect. Neutralization experiment using anti-AM antibody revealed a marked enhancement of endothelial apoptosis after serum starvation. Since AM is synthesized by and secreted from RAEC in an autocrine/paracrine manner, our data are consistent with the notion that autocrine-secreted endogenous AM functions as a survival factor for endothelial cells (Kato et al., 1997). In spite of cAMP response by AM in RAECs, cAMP antagonist (Rp-cAMPS) failed to inhibit, and cAMP-elevating agonists (forskolin, PGI_2) could not mimic, the anti-apoptotic effect by AM (Kato et al., 1997), suggesting that AM exerts its anti-apoptotic effect through the mechanism independent of cAMP/PKA pathway.

Then, we clarified the molecular mechanism of anti-apoptotic action by AM

(Shichiri et al., 1999). Myc is recognized as one of the key proto-oncogenes regulating cell cycle progression and cell proliferation, while it can promote apoptosis in the absence of survival factor (Pelengaris et al., 2002). Myc, when heterodimerized with its binding partner, Max, exerts transcriptional activity on its target genes through binding to its cognate DNA binding site (E-box), whereas both Max-Max homodimer and heterodimer with alternative partner (Mad, Mxi) can also bind to E-box, but do not show any transcriptional activity on the target gene, thus Myc functioning as a transcriptional repressor (Pelengaris et al., 2002; Yin et al., 1998). In serum-starved quiescent RAECs, AM upregulates Max gene expression without affecting Myc gene expression, thereby leading to the increased Max/Myc ratio. In addition, overexpression of Max gene mimicked the anti-apoptotic effect of AM in serum-starved RAEC, whose effect was abrogated by antisense oligonucleotides against Max (Shichiri et al., 1999). Collectively, these data clearly demonstrates that AM exerts its anti-apoptotic effect through the upregulation of Max gene to block the c-Myc-mediated apoptosis independently from cAMP/PKA pathway (Fig. 4).

Subsequently, the anti-apoptotic effect by AM has been reported in various cell types, including endometrial cancer cells (Oehler et al., 2001), human adrenal zonna glomerulosa cells (Rebuffat et al., 2002), human skin keratinocyte and fibroblast (Albertin et al., 2003). However, the biological significance of the anti-apoptotic effect by AM has not been fully understood. Recent gene targeting experiments of AM gene reveals that the AM null mice are embryonic lethal due to the abnormal development of cardiovascular system (Shindo et al., 2001). Thus endothelial anti-apoptotic effect by AM may play an integral role in embryogenesis, especially cardiovascular development.

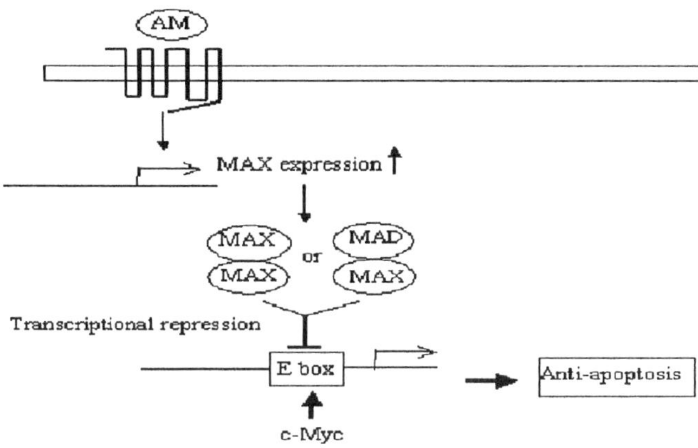

Fig. 4 The mechanism of anti-apoptotic action by AM
AM upregulates MAX expression, but not that of c-MYC, which results in increase in MAX/MYC ratio. This relative excess of MAX leads to predominant formation of MAX-MAX and MAD-MAX dimers rather than MYC-MAX, which function as E-box transcriptional repressor, thereby leading to anti-apoptotic effect.

(2) ANTI-MIGRATION EFFECT

The effect of AM on cell migration has been studied in VSMCs using Boyden chamber (Horio T et al., 1995; Kohno M et al., 1997; Kohno M et al., 1999). In these studies, AM has been shown to inhibit serum-, Ang II-, and PDGF-stimulated VSMC migration. The mechanism of anti-migratory effect by AM appears to be mediated in cAMP/PKA pathway, since its anti-migratory effect as accompanied by cAMP response, and cAMP-elevating agonists (8-bromo cAMP, forskolin, PGI_2) mimicked the effect.
We investigated the differential role of CRLR/RAMP system in the anti-migratory effect using monolayer-wounding of rat VSMC and fibroblasts (Fukai et al., 2003). AM potently exhibited the anti-migratory effect in VSMC where CRLR and RAMP isoforms (1, 2, 3) were co-expressed,

whereas it did not show any effect in fibroblasts where CRLR and RAMP1, but not RAMP2/3, were co-expressed. Failure of CGRP to induce anti-migratory response in VSMC and fibroblasts strongly suggests that the anti-migratory effect is mediated via a specific AM receptors comprising CRLR/RAMP2 or 3. Furthermore, co-transfection of RAMP2 or RAMP3 with CRLR revealed slower cell migration in VSMC and fibroblasts, whose effect was further enhanced by AM. Thus specific AM receptor consisting of both CRLR and RAMP (2, 3) mediates AM-induced anti-migratory response. However, cAMP-elevating agonists failed to mimic, and cAMP antagonist could not block the anti-migratory effect by AM. Furthermore, any of several inhibitors for well-known signaling molecules, such as cGMP, ERK, p38 MAPK, PTK, and PI3 kinase, all failed to block the anti-migratory response by AM. Thus molecular mechanisms of anti-migratory response by AM other than cAMP/PKA pathway remains to be determined (Fukai et al., 2003). The reasons for the apparent discrepancy between our results and those of previous studies could be accounted for by the different experimental methods (wound healing vs. Boyden chamber).

CONCLUDING REMARKS

Expression of AM and its receptor has been shown to be not confined to cardiovascular system, but widely and ubiquitously distributed in variety of tissues. Since its discovery as a potent vasodilator, there have been extensive investigations revealing pleiotropic effects of AM. Recent discovery of CRLR/RAMP system that confers ligand selectivity for AM and CGRP facilitates the understanding of new-facet of AM/CGRP receptors and their signaling pathways. However, further characterization of CRLR/RAMP system is required to connect the missing link between molecular mechanism and experimental data of pleiotropic functions by AM. Development of receptor antagonists highly selective for AM with higher-affinity and their application in experimental and clinical settings could help the understanding of complex pharmacology of AM *in vivo*.

REFERENCES

Aiyar N, Rand K, Elshourbagy N A, Zeng Z, Adamou JE, Bergsma, DJ, and Li Y (1996) A cDNA encoding the calcitonin gene-related peptide type 1 receptor. J Biol Chem 271:11325-11329.

Albertin G, Carraro G, Parnigotto PP, Conconi MT, Ziolkowska A, Malendowicz LK, and Nussdorfer GG (2003) Human skin keratinocytes and fibroblasts express adrenomedullin and its receptors, and adrenomedullin enhances their growth in vitro by stimulating proliferation and inhibiting apoptosis. Int J Mol Med 11:635-639.

Aldecoa A, Gujer R, Fischer JA, and Born W (2000) Mammalian calcitonin receptor-like receptor/receptor activity modifying protein complexes define calcitonin gene-related peptide and adrenomedullin receptors in Drosophila Schneider 2 cells. FEBS Lett 471:156-160.

Benovic JL, Pike LJ, Cerione RA, Staniszewski C, Yoshimasa T, Codina J, Caron MG, and Lefkowitz RJ. (1985) Phosphorylation of the mammalian beta-adrenergic receptor by cyclic AMP-dependent protein kinase. Regulation of the rate of receptor phosphorylation and dephosphorylation by agonist occupancy and effects on coupling of the receptor to the stimulatory guanine nucleotide regulatory protein. J Biol Chem 260:7094-7101.

Born W, Muff R, and Fischer JA. (2002) Functional interaction of G protein-coupled receptors of the adrenomedullin peptide family with accessory receptor-activity-modifying proteins (RAMP). Microsc Res Tech 57:14-22.

Chini EN, Choi E, Grande JP, Burnett JC, and Dousa TP. (1995) Adrenomedullin suppresses mitogenesis in rat mesangial cells via cAMP pathway. Biochem Biophys Res Commun 215:868-873.

Christopoulos G, Perry KJ, Morfis M, Tilakaratne N, Gao Y, Fraser NJ, Main MJ, Foord SM, and Sexton PM. (1999) Multiple amylin receptors arise from receptor activity-modifying protein interaction with the calcitonin receptor gene product. Mol Pharmacol 56:235-242.

Coppock HA, Owji AA, Bloom SR, and Smith DM. (1996) A rat skeletal muscle cell line (L6) expresses specific adrenomedullin binding sites but activates adenylate cyclase via calcitonin gene-related peptide receptors. Biochem J 318:241-245.

Eguchi S, Hirata Y, Iwasaki H, Sato K, Watanabe TX, Inui T, Nakajima K, Sakakibara S, and Marumo F. (1994a) Structure-activity relationship of adrenomedullin, a novel vasodilatory peptide, in cultured rat vascular smooth muscle cells. Endocrinology 135:2454-2458.

Eguchi S, Hirata Y, Kano H, Sato K, Watanabe Y, Watanabe TX, Nakajima K, Sakakibara S, and Marumo F. (1994b) Specific receptors for adrenomedullin in cultured rat vascular smooth muscle cells. FEBS Lett 340:226-230.

Elshourbagy NA, Adamou JE, Swift AM, Disa J, Mao J, Ganguly S, Bergsma DJ, and Aiyar N. (1998) Molecular cloning and characterization of the porcine calcitonin gene-related peptide receptor. Endocrinology 139:1678-1683.

Entzeroth M, Doods HN, Wieland HA, and Wienen W. (1995) Adrenomedullin

mediates vasodilation via CGRP1 receptors. Life Sci 56:PL19-25.
Evans BN, Rosenblatt MI, Mnayer LO, Oliver KR, and Dickerson IM. (2000) CGRP-RCP, a novel protein required for signal transduction at calcitonin gene-related peptide and adrenomedullin receptors. J Biol Chem 275:31438-31443.
Flahaut M, Rossier BC, and Firsov D. (2002) Respective roles of calcitonin receptor-like receptor (CRLR) and receptor activity-modifying proteins (RAMP) in cell surface expression of CRLR/RAMP heterodimeric receptors. J Biol Chem 277:14731-14737.
Fluhmann B, Muff R, Hunziker W, Fischer JA, and Born W. (1995) A human orphan calcitonin receptor-like structure. Biochem Biophys Res Commun 206:341-347.
Fukai N, Shichiri M, Ozawa N, Matsushita M, and Hirata Y. (2003) Coexpression of calcitonin receptor-like receptor and receptor activity-modifying protein 2 or 3 mediates the antimigratory effect of adrenomedullin. Endocrinology 144:447-453.
Gether U. (2000) Uncovering molecular mechanisms involved in activation of G protein-coupled receptors. Endocr Rev 21:90-113.
Hall JM, Siney L, Lippton H, Hyman A, Kang-Chang J, and Brain SD. (1995) Interaction of human adrenomedullin 13-52 with calcitonin gene-related peptide receptors in the microvasculature of the rat and hamster. Br J Pharmacol 114:592-597.
Han ZQ, Coppock HA, Smith DM, Van Noorden S, Makgoba MW, Nicholl CG, and Legon S. (1997) The interaction of CGRP and adrenomedullin with a receptor expressed in the rat pulmonary vascular endothelium. J Mol Endocrinol 18:267-272.
Hausdorff WP, Bouvier M, O'Dowd BF, Irons GP, Caron MG, and Lefkowitz RJ. (1989) Phosphorylation sites on two domains of the beta 2-adrenergic receptor are involved in distinct pathways of receptor desensitization. J Biol Chem 264:12657-12665.
Hilairet S, Foord SM, Marshall FH, and Bouvier M. (2001) Protein-protein interaction and not glycosylation determines the binding selectivity of heterodimers between the calcitonin receptor-like receptor and the receptor activity-modifying proteins. J Biol Chem 276:29575-29581.
Hinson JP, Kapas S, and Smith DM. (2000) Adrenomedullin, a multifunctional regulatory peptide. Endocr Rev 21:138-167.
Hirata Y, Mitaka C, Sato K, Nagura T, Tsunoda Y, Amaha K, and Marumo F. (1996) Increased circulating adrenomedullin, a novel vasodilatory peptide, in sepsis. J Clin Endocrinol Metab 81:1449-1453.
Horio T, Kohno M, Kano H, Ikeda M, Yasunari K, Yokokawa K, Minami M, and Takeda T. (1995) Adrenomedullin as a novel antimigration factor of vascular smooth muscle cells. Circ Res 77:660-664.
Ishiyama Y, Kitamura K, Ichiki Y, Nakamura S, Kida O, Kangawa K, and Eto T.

(1993) Hemodynamic effects of a novel hypotensive peptide, human adrenomedullin, in rats. Eur J Pharmacol 241:271-273.

Iwasaki H, Eguchi S, Shichiri M, Marumo F, and Hirata Y. (1998a) Adrenomedullin as a novel growth-promoting factor for cultured vascular smooth muscle cells: role of tyrosine kinase-mediated mitogen-activated protein kinase activation. Endocrinology 139:3432-3441.

Iwasaki H, Eguchi S, Shichiri M, Marumo F, and Hirata Y. (1998b) Down-regulation of adenylate cyclase coupled to adrenomedullin receptor in vascular smooth muscle cells. Eur J Pharmacol 352:131-134.

Iwasaki H, Shichiri M, Marumo F, and Hirata Y. (2001) Adrenomedullin stimulates proline-rich tyrosine kinase 2 in vascular smooth muscle cells. Endocrinology 142:564-572.

Kano H, Kohno M, Yasunari K, Yokokawa K, Horio T, Ikeda M, Minami M, Hanehira T, Takeda T, and Yoshikawa J. (1996) Adrenomedullin as a novel antiproliferative factor of vascular smooth muscle cells. J Hypertens 14:209-213.

Kapas S, Brown DW, Farthing PM, and Hagi-Pavli E. (1997) Adrenomedullin has mitogenic effects on human oral keratinocytes: involvement of cyclic AMP. FEBS Lett 418:287-290.

Kato H, Shichiri M, Marumo F, and Hirata Y. (1997) Adrenomedullin as an autocrine/paracrine apoptosis survival factor for rat endothelial cells. Endocrinology 138:2615-2620.

Kim W, Moon SO, Sung MJ, Kim SH, Lee S, So JN, and Park SK. (2003) Angiogenic role of adrenomedullin through activation of Akt, mitogen-activated protein kinase, and focal adhesion kinase in endothelial cells. FASEB J 17:1937-1939.

Kitamura K, Kangawa K, and Eto T. (2002) Adrenomedullin and PAMP: discovery, structures, and cardiovascular functions. Microsc Res Tech 57:3-13.

Kitamura K, Kangawa K, Kawamoto M, Ichiki Y, Nakamura S, Matsuo H, and Eto T. (1993) Adrenomedullin: a novel hypotensive peptide isolated from human pheochromocytoma. Biochem Biophys Res Commun 192:553-560.

Kohno M, Yokokawa K, Kano H, Yasunari K, Minami M, Hanehira T, and Yoshikawa J. (1997) Adrenomedullin is a potent inhibitor of angiotensin II-induced migration of human coronary artery smooth muscle cells. Hypertension 29:1309-1313.

Kohno M, Yasunari K, Minami M, Kano H, Maeda K, Mandel AK, Inoki K, Haneda M, and Yoshikawa J. (1999) Regulation of rat mesangial cell migration by platelet-derived growth factor, angiotensin II, and adrenomedullin. J Am Soc Nephrol 10:2495-2502.

Leuthauser K, Gujer R, Aldecoa A, McKinney RA, Muff R, Fischer JA, and Born W. (2000) Receptor-activity-modifying protein 1 forms heterodimers with two G-protein-coupled receptors to define ligand recognition. Biochem J 351:347-351.

Lin HY, Harris TL, Flannery MS, Aruffo A, Kaji EH, Gorn A, Kolakowski LF Jr., Lodish HF, and Goldring SR. (1991) Expression cloning of an adenylate cyclase-coupled calcitonin receptor. Science 254:1022-1024.

Luebke AE, Dahl GP, Roos BA, and Dickerson IM. (1996) Identification of a protein that confers calcitonin gene-related peptide responsiveness to oocytes by using a cystic fibrosis transmembrane conductance regulator assay. Proc Natl Acad Sci U S A 93:3455-3460.

Martinez A, Elsasser TH, Muro-Cacho C, Moody TW, Miller MJ, Macri CJ, and Cuttitta F. (1997) Expression of adrenomedullin and its receptor in normal and malignant human skin: a potential pluripotent role in the integument. Endocrinology 138:5597-5604.

McLatchie LM, Fraser NJ, Main MJ, Wise A, Brown J, Thompson N, Solari R, Lee MG, and Foord SM. (1998) RAMPs regulate the transport and ligand specificity of the calcitonin-receptor-like receptor. Nature 393:333-339.

Miller MJ, Martinez A, Unsworth EJ, Thiele CJ, Moody TW, Elsasser T, and Cuttitta F. (1996) Adrenomedullin expression in human tumor cell lines. Its potential role as an autocrine growth factor. J Biol Chem 271:23345-23351.

Muff R, Buhlmann N, Fischer JA, and Born W. (1999) An amylin receptor is revealed following co-transfection of a calcitonin receptor with receptor activity modifying proteins-1 or -3. Endocrinology 140: 2924-2927.

Nishimatsu H, Suzuki E, Nagata D, Moriyama N, Satonaka H, Walsh K, Sata M, Kangawa K, Matsuo H, Goto A, Kitamura T, and Hirata Y. (2001) Adrenomedullin induces endothelium-dependent vasorelaxation via the phosphatidylinositol 3-kinase/Akt-dependent pathway in rat aorta. Circ Res 89:63-70.

Njuki F, Nicholl CG, Howard A, Mak JC, Barnes PJ, Girgis SI, and Legon S. (1993) A new calcitonin-receptor-like sequence in rat pulmonary blood vessels. Clin Sci (Lond) 85:385-388.

Nuki C, Kawasaki H, Kitamura K, Takenaga M, Kangawa K, Eto T, and Wada A. (1993) Vasodilator effect of adrenomedullin and calcitonin gene-related peptide receptors in rat mesenteric vascular beds. Biochem Biophys Res Commun 196:245-251.

Nussdorfer GG, Rossi GP, and Mazzocchi G. (1997) Role of adrenomedullin and related peptides in the regulation of the hypothalamo-pituitary-adrenal axis. Peptides 18:1079-1089.

Oehler MK, Norbury C, Hague S, Rees MC, and Bicknell R. (2001) Adrenomedullin inhibits hypoxic cell death by upregulation of Bcl-2 in endometrial cancer cells: a possible promotion mechanism for tumour growth. Oncogene 20:2937-2945.

Okumura H, Nagaya N, Itoh T, Okano I, Hino J, Mori K, Tsukamoto Y, Ishibashi-Ueda H, Miwa S, Tambara K, Toyokuni S, Yunati C, and Kangawa K.

(2004) Adrenomedullin infusion attenuates myocardial ischemia/reperfusion injury through the phosphatidylinositol 3-kinase/Akt-dependent pathway. Circulation 109:242-248.

Owji AA, Gardiner JV, Upton PD, Mahmoodi M, Ghatei MA, Bloom SR, and Smith DM. (1996) Characterisation and molecular identification of adrenomedullin binding sites in the rat spinal cord: a comparison with calcitonin gene-related peptide receptors. J Neurochem 67:2172-2179.

Owji AA, Smith DM, Coppock HA, Morgan DG, Bhogal R, Ghatei MA, and Bloom SR. (1995) An abundant and specific binding site for the novel vasodilator adrenomedullin in the rat. Endocrinology 136:2127-2134.

Parkes DG, and May CN. (1997) Direct cardiac and vascular actions of adrenomedullin in conscious sheep. Br J Pharmacol 120:1179-1185.

Pelengaris S, Khan M, and Evan G. (2002) c-MYC: more than just a matter of life and death. Nat Rev Cancer 2:764-776.

Poyner DR, Sexton P M, Marshall I, Smith DM, Quirion R, Born W, Muff R, Fischer JA, and Foord SM. (2002) International Union of Pharmacology. XXXII. The mammalian calcitonin gene-related peptides, adrenomedullin, amylin, and calcitonin receptors. Pharmacol Rev 54:233-246.

Prado MA, Evans-Bain B, Oliver KR, and Dickerson IM. (2001) The role of the CGRP-receptor component protein (RCP) in adrenomedullin receptor signal transduction. Peptides 22:1773-1781.

Rebuffat P, Forneris ML, Aragona F, Ziolkowska A, Malendowicz LK, and Nussdorfer GG. (2002) Adrenomedullin and its receptors are expressed in the zona glomerulosa of human adrenal gland: evidence that ADM enhances proliferation and decreases apoptosis in cultured ZG cells. Int J Mol Med 9:119-124.

Segawa K, Minami K, Sata T, Kuroiwa A, and Shigematsu A. (1996) Inhibitory effect of adrenomedullin on rat mesangial cell mitogenesis. Nephron 74:577-579.

Shichiri M, Fukai N, Ozawa N, Iwasaki H, and Hirata Y. (2003) Adrenomedullin is an autocrine/paracrine growth factor for rat vascular smooth muscle cells. Regul Pept 112:167-173.

Shichiri M, and Hirata Y. (2003) Regulation of cell growth and apoptosis by adrenomedullin. Hypertens Res 26:S9-14.

Shichiri M, Kato H, Doi M, Marumo F, and Hirata Y. (1999) Induction of max by adrenomedullin and calcitonin gene-related peptide antagonizes endothelial apoptosis. Mol Endocrinol 13:1353-1363.

Shimekake Y, Nagata K, Ohta S, Kambayashi Y, Teraoka H, Kitamura K, Eto T, Kangawa K, and Matsuo H. (1995) Adrenomedullin stimulates two signal transduction pathways, cAMP accumulation and Ca^{2+} mobilization, in bovine aortic endothelial cells. J Biol Chem 270:4412-4417.

Shimosawa T, Shibasaki Y, Ishibashi K, Kitamura K, Kangawa K, Kato S, Ando K, and Fujita T. (2002) Adrenomedullin, an endogenous peptide, counteracts cardiovascular damage. Circulation 105:106-111.

Shindo T, Kurihara Y, Nishimatsu H, Moriyama N, Kakoki M, Wang Y, Imai Y, Ebihara A, Kuwaki T, Ju KH, Minamino N, Kangawa K, Ishikawa T, Fukuda M, Akimoto Y, Kawakami H, Imai T, Morita H, Yazaki Y, Nagai R, Hirata Y, and Kurihara H. (2001) Vascular abnormalities and elevated blood pressure in mice lacking adrenomedullin gene. Circulation 104:1964-1971.

Sugo S, Minamino N, Shoji H, Kangawa K, Kitamura K, Eto T, and Matsuo H. (1995) Interleukin-1, tumor necrosis factor and lipopolysaccharide additively stimulate production of adrenomedullin in vascular smooth muscle cells. Biochem Biophys Res Commun 207:25-32.

Takahashi K, Satoh F, Hara E, Murakami O, Kumabe T, Tominaga T, Kayama T, Yoshimoto T, and Shibahara S. (1997a) Production and secretion of adrenomedullin by cultured choroid plexus carcinoma cells. J Neurochem 68:726-731.

Takahashi K, Satoh F, Hara E, Sone M, Murakami O, Kayama T, Yoshimoto T, and Shibahara S. (1997b) Production and secretion of adrenomedullin from glial cell tumors and its effects on cAMP production. Peptides 18:1117-1124.

Togawa M, Haneda M, Araki S, Sugimoto T, Isono M, Hidaka H, Yasuda H, Kashiwagi A, and Kikkawa R. (1997) Beraprost sodium, an analogue of prostacyclin, induces the expression of mitogen-activated protein kinase phosphatase and inhibits the proliferation of cultured mesangial cells. Eur J Pharmacol 336:291-294.

Wang HY, Hadcock JR, and Malbon CC. (1990) Beta-adrenergic receptor regulation. New insights on biochemical and molecular mechanisms. Receptor 1:13-32.

Withers DJ., Coppock HA., Seufferlein T, Smith DM, Bloom SR, and Rozengurt E. (1996) Adrenomedullin stimulates DNA synthesis and cell proliferation via elevation of cAMP in Swiss 3T3 cells. FEBS Lett 378:83-87.

Yin H, Chao L, and Chao J. (2004) Adrenomedullin protects against myocardial apoptosis after ischemia/reperfusion through activation of Akt-GSK signaling. Hypertension 43:109-116.

Yin X, Grove L, and Prochownik EV. (1998) Lack of transcriptional repression by max homodimers. Oncogene 16:2629-2637.

Yoshimoto T, Fukai N, Sato R, Sugiyama T, Ozawa N, Shichiri M, and Hirata Y. (2004) Anti-oxidant effect of adrenomedullin on angiotensin II-induced ROS generation in vascular smooth muscle cells. Endocrinology 145:3331-3337.

Zimmermann U, Fischer JA, and Muff R. (1995) Adrenomedullin and calcitonin gene-related peptide interact with the same receptor in cultured human neuroblastoma SK-N-MC cells. Peptides 16:421-424.

3

ADRENOMEDULLIN GENE

Toshihiko Ishimitsu, Kohju Tsukada, Junichi Minami, Hidehiko Ono, and Hiroaki Matsuoka

Department of Hypertension and Cardiorenal Medicine, Dokkyo University School of Medicine, Mibu, Tochigi 321-0293, Japan

INTRODUCTION

Adrenomedullin (AM) is a vasodilator peptide originally discovered in pheochromocytoma tissue by Kitamura et al. (Kitamura et al., 1993a). However, the mRNA of AM has been shown to be expressed not only in the adrenal gland but also in various cardiovascular organs, such as the heart, kidney and blood vessels (Kitamura et al., 1993b). Furthermore, it has been demonstrated that a significant level of AM exists in the circulating human plasma (Kitamura et al., 1994a). We have also reported that plasma AM levels are increased in patients with various cardiovascular diseases, such as hypertension, heart failure and renal failure (Ishimitsu et al., 1994a; Nishikimi et al., 1995). Thus, it is suggested that AM has a significant role in the pathophysiology of cardiovascular system.

In order to clarify the roles of AM in the cardiovascular system, it is essential to analyze the structure and the function of the human AM gene. Especially, the analysis of the 5'-flanking region of the genomic gene provides information as to the regulatory mechanism of the gene transcription. In addition, if there is inter-individual variation in the DNA nucleotide sequences of the human AM gene, the variation may be related to the function of the AM gene and the pathogenesis of cardiovascular disorders. In this chapter, we survey the results of studies concerning the analysis of human AM gene and its relation to the pathophysiology of cardiovascular diseases.

1. GENOMIC STRUCTURE OF THE HUMAN AM GENE

The cDNA sequence of the human AM gene was reported by Kitamura et al.

(Kitamura et al., 1993b). We have previously cloned the genomic DNA encoding the human AM gene from a human liver genomic library constructed in charon 4A λ phages by the plaque hybridization method using human AM cDNA as the probe (Ishimitsu et al., 1994b). The DNA nucleotide sequence was then determined by a dideoxynucleotide chain terminating method and urea-polyacrylamide gel electrophoresis. As shown in Figure 1, the gene is composed of four exons interposed by three introns. The whole nucleotide sequence corresponding to the 52 amino acid residues of the mature AM is included in the fourth exon, and the nucleotides of proadrenomedullin N-terminal 20 peptide (PAMP), another bioactive peptide produced from AM mRNA (Kitamura et al., 1994b), spread over the second and third exons.

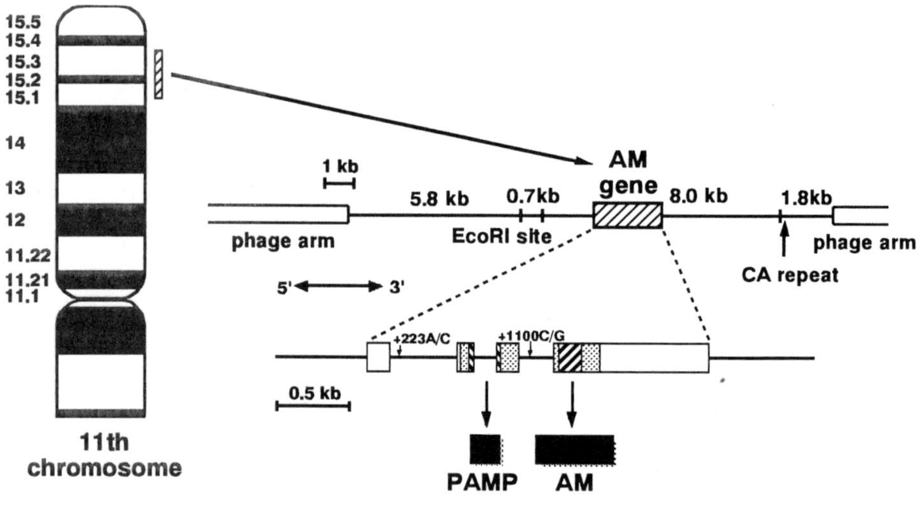

Figure 1. Genomic organization of human AM gene. Dotted area within the exons are translated into the peptide, proadrenomedullin. The heavily hatched area corresponds to mature AM and the proadrenomedullin N-terminal 20 peptide (PAMP).

Southern blot analysis of the DNA from 20 human-hamster somatic cell lines carrying certain human chromosomes was performed using the cloned genomic DNA fragment encoding the human AM gene as a probe (Ishimitsu et al., 1994b). The labeled probe DNA was hybridized only with the DNA from cell lines containing human chromosome 11 (Ishimitsu et al., 1994b). Therefore, it was determined that the human AM gene is localized on chromosome 11. Further chromosomal sublocalization of the human AM gene was performed with the fluorescence *in situ* hybridization (FISH) technique (Ishimitsu et al., 2001). The cultured human lymphocytes treated with BrdU for synchronization were fixed on slides and hybridized with a fluorescence-labeled genomic DNA fragment encoding the human AM gene in full length. The fluorescent signal from the probe was detected on the distal end of the short arm of chromosome 11. Thus, the human AM gene was located at chromosome 11 (Ishimitsu et al., 2001), region p15.1-3, as depicted in Figure 1. Near the location of human AM gene, There exist several other known genes, such as sphingomyelinase (p15.1-4), parathyroid hormone (p15.1-2) and lactate dehydrogenase (p14-15.1) (da Veiga Pereira et al., 1991; Arnold et al., 1989; Li et al., 1988).

2. PROMOTER ACTIVITY OF 5'-FLANKING REGION OF HUMAN AM GENE

Besides the adrenal gland, the mRNA of AM is widely expressed in cardiovascular tissues. The cultured cells such as fibroblasts, vascular endothelial cells and smooth muscle cells have been shown to express AM mRNA prominently (Sugo et al., 1994a; Sugo et al., 1994b; Tomoda et al., 2001). We examined the promoter activity of the human AM gene in cultured human aortic endothelial cells (HAEC) (Ishimitsu et al., 1998). First, the transcription start site was determined by the primer extension method using total RNA extracted from HAEC as the template. As framed in Figure 2, two transcription start sites were identified, both at the cytosine nucleotides. These are 21 and 25 bases downstream from the TATA box and 19 and 23 bases upstream from the 5'-end of the human AM cDNA sequence determined by Kitamura et al. (Kitamura et al., 1993b). Hereafter, the upstream transcription start site at nucleotide C is assigned the nucleotide number 1.

```
-150  CCAACTCCAG CCCCAAAGGA AGCAATGCGC GCGTCCGAGA GCAGGAGCGC

               NF-IL6                         AP-2        AP-2
-100  GCGTGGCTGA GGAAAGAAAG GGAAGGCAAC CGGGCAGCCC AGGCCCCGCC
                                                 AP-2       AP-2

                  AP-2
       AP-2       AP-2
-50   CCGCCGCTCC CCCACCCGTG CGCTTATAAA GCACAGGAAC CAGAGCTGGC
                  AP-2
                  AP-2

 +1   GACTGAGTGG TTTCTTGGTG ACACTGGATA
```

Figure 2. Nucleotide sequence of the promoter region of human AM gene. Two transcription start sites (+1 and +5) are framed and the TATA box is underlined. NF-IL6 nuclear factor for interleukin-6 expression; AP-2, activator protein 2.

Next, the genomic DNA fragment corresponding to nucleotide positions –1534 to +70 from the transcription start site was ligated into the luciferase reporter vector. The plasmid was conjugated with liposome and transfected into cultured HAEC. The promoter activity of the inserted DNA was evaluated by measuring the expressed luciferase activity using a luminometer. When the length of the inserted DNA was gradually shortened by exonuclease III and mung bean nuclease digestion from the 5'-end, the expressed luciferase activity was decreased by 41% in the absence of nucleotides –110 to –90 and then was further decreased by 42% in the absence of nucleotides –66 to –29.

Figure 3 shows the distribution of the consensus sequences of binding sites for transcription factors. There is a consensus sequence of the nuclear factor for the interleukin-6 expression (NF-IL6) binding site (TGAGGAAAG) at nucleotides –93 to –85 of the human AM gene, and nucleotides –68 to –32 contain multiple binding sites for activator protein 2 (AP-2). When the NF-IL6 consensus sequence was mutated to TGAGtActG, the promoter activity to express luciferase was reduced by 42%. Furthermore, the electrophoretic mobility shift assay revealed that the nuclear extract from HAEC contains a protein binding to the AP-2 consensus oligonucleotide. Thus, it is suggested that the two transcription factors, NF-IL6 and AP-2, participate in the regulation of basal expression of the human AM gene in vascular endothelial cells.

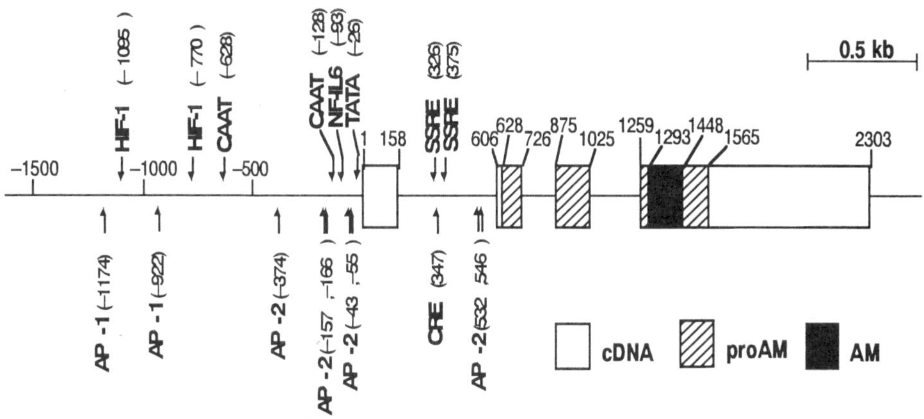

Figure 3. Distribution of consensus sequences for binding sites of transcription factors in the promoter region of the human adrenomedullin gene. AP-1, activator protein 1; AP-2, activator protein 2; HIF-1, hypoxia-inducible factor-1; CAAT, CAAT box; TATA, TATA box; NF-IL6, nuclear factor for interleukin-6 expression; SSRE, shear stress responsive element; CRE, cAMP responsive element.

3. FACTORS REGULATING AM GENE EXPRESSION

(1) Inflammatory Cytokines and NO

In vitro experiments using cultured cells have indicated that the production of AM is increased by the stimulation of cytokines such as inteleukin-1 (IL-1) and tumor necrosis factor-α (TNF-α) (Isumi et al., 1998). In clinical settings as well, plasma AM has been shown to be markedly elevated in patients with infectious or inflammatory disorders (Ishimitsu et al., 1999; Hirata et al., 1996). Considering that NF-IL6 has been shown to be induced by stimulation with IL-1, TNF-α and IL-6 itself, NF-IL6 may partly mediate these increases in AM induced by cytokines. In the acute-phase reaction against inflammation or tissue injury, NF-IL6 is assumed to play an important role as a transcription factor. It is speculated that AM, induced by NF-IL6, dilates regional blood vessels and facilitates the delivery of blood and leukocytes to the inflamed tissue. On the other hand, it has been reported that nitric oxide (NO), the endothelium-derived vasorelaxing factor, promotes the expression of AM mRNA in vascular endothelial and smooth muscle cells, and thereby mediating the actions of inflammatory cytokines (Hofbauer et al., 2002).

(2) Ischemia, Hypoxia and Oxidative Stress

Multiple lines of evidence indicate that hypoxia or oxidative stress induces AM mRNA expression (Cormier-Regard et al., 1998; Ladoux et al., 2000; Ogita et al., 2001; Chun et al., 2000), and Cormier-Regard et al. have reported that the hypoxia-inducible factor-1 (HIF-1) consensus binding site locating at nucleotide position –1095 of the mouse AM gene mediates this hypoxia-induced AM gene expression (Cormier-Regard et al., 1998). The 5'-flanking region of the human AM gene also contains this HIF-1 consensus sequence at nucleotides –825, -863 and –1203. It has been also reported that endothelial PAS domain protein 1 (EPAS1), which plays an important role in the gene expressions induced by hypoxic stimuli, promotes AM gene expression via Src, a non-receptor tyrosine kinase, in cardiomyocytes (Tanaka et al., 2002). This pathway has been shown to be common with the signal transduction system of inflammatory stimuli such as IL-1. As to the pathophysiological implication of AM induced by ischemia and hypoxia, Wang *et al.* have reported that AM mRNA expression is increased by focal ischemic injury in the rat brain cortex (Wang et al., 1995). Thus, the increased AM may dilate focal blood vessels and thereby serve to restore blood flow to the ischemic tissue.

(3) Mechanical and Physical Stimuli

We and other groups have reported that plasma AM is increased in patients with hypertension (Ishimitsu et al., 1994a; Kato et al., 1999; Kohno et al., 1996), and acute pressure overload has been shown to stimulate left ventricular AM gene expression in rats (Romppanen et al., 1997). In the *ex vivo* experiment, Ruskoaho et al (Luodonpaa et al., 2003) have reported that acute pressure loading increases the AM gene expression in the left ventricle using the isolated perfused heart of rat, however, stretching of cultured neonatal ventricular myocytes resulted in inhibition of AM gene expression. On the contrary, Tsuruda et al (Tsuruda et al., 2000) have observed enhanced AM gene expression and secretion by mechanical stretching in cultured rat cardiomyocytes. Conflicting results have been also reported as to the effect of shear stress on AM mRNA expression in cultured endothelial cells (Chun et al., 1997; Shinoki et al., 1998). Namely, Chun et al have reported the increase in AM mRNA expression by shear stress in cultured endothelial cells of human umbilical vein, while Shinoki et al have observed rather suppressive effect of physiological shear stress on the AM mRNA expression in HAEC. In any way, considering that there are two consensus sequences of the shear stress responsive element in the intron 1 human AM gene (Figure 3), it is possible that transcription of the AM gene is affected by physical and mechanical stimuli.

(4) Interactions with Other Neuroendocrine Factors

With regard to the role of AP-2 in the regulation of AM gene transcription, Nakayama *et al.* have also reported that phorbol ester, an agonist of diacylglycerol (DAG), induces AM gene expression in human monocytic leukemia cells, and the cis-acting region (-70 to –30) containing multiple AP-2 binding sites is necessary for this induction (Nakayama et al., 2000). As already mentioned, plasma AM is increased in patients with hypertension, heart failure and renal failure (Ishimitsu et al., 1994a; Nishikimi et al., 1995; Kato et al., 1999). In the process of cardiovascular disease development, cardiovascular neuroendocrine systems such as the sympathetic nerve system and renin-angiotensin system are activated. Stimulations of α_1-adrenergic receptor and type 1 angiotensin II (AII) receptor both elicit activation of phospholipase C (PLC), production of DAG, activation of protein kinase C (PKC) and induction of AP-2. This pathway may be involved in the mechanism of increased plasma AM in various cardiovascular diseases. Indeed, it has been reported that PKC and Ca^{2+}/calmodulin signaling system are involved in AII-induced AM secretion from rat cardiac myocytes (Tsuruda et al., 2001). Also in *in vivo* study and in clinical patients, ACE inhibition was shown to reduce cardiac AM gene expression in dogs with congestive heart failure (Jougasaki et al., 2001) and plasma AM concentrations were shown to be high in patients with high-renin essential hypertension (Letizia et al., 2002).

On the other hand, Barker et al. have suggested that a protein kinase other than PKC is involved in the regulation of AM mRNA production by bovine aortic endothelial cells (Barker et al., 1998). Furthermore, Autelitano *et al.* have indicated that phorbor ester and PKC activation inhibit, rather than promoting, AM gene expression by neonatal rat cardiomyocytes (Autelitano et al., 2001). Although the effect of AP-2 may differ according to the species and the cell types, AP-2 is thought to participate in the transcriptional regulation of the AM gene.

AM is known to stimulate cAMP production in various cells, and cAMP is thought to serve as a second messenger of the biological actions of AM. On the other hand, AM gene expression has been shown to be decreased by cAMP (Sugo et al., 1995; Kobayashi et al., 1999). Although it has not yet been proven, the consensus sequence of the cAMP responsive element existing in intron 1 at the nuclotide position of +347 may transmit this negative feedback signal.

Steroid hormones are also supposed to affect production of AM. It has been reported that aldosterone, a mineralocorticoid, augments AM gene expression in cultured human aortic smooth muscle cells (Uemura et al., 2002). On the other hand, dexamethasone, a glucocorticoid, has been shown to suppress the expression of AM gene in human glioblastoma cells (Takahashi et al., 2003). Estrogen and its receptor are supposed to affect AM gene expressions in the ovary and uterus (Giacalone et al., 2003; Cameron et al., 2002), however, the AM gene expression in the prostate tissue was shown to be androgen-independent (Jimenez et al., 2003).

With regard to other endocrine factors, plasma AM concentrations were observed to be elevated in patients with hyperparathyroidism (Letizia et al., 2003) and acute hyperinsulinemia was shown to increase plasma AM in patients with type 2 diabetes (Katsuki et al., 2002). In experiments using cultured human skin and oral keratinocytes, endothelin-1 has shown to increase adrenomedullin production (Kapas et al., 2001). These suggest the influence of insulin, endothelin and parathyroid hormone on AM gene expression.

(5) Oncogenes and Carcinogens

It has been shown that several tumor cells express AM mRNA and produce AM (Udono et al., 2000; Dotsch et al., 2000; Hata et al., 2000; Rocchi et al., 2001). AM has been shown to induce expression of Max which forms a

heterodimer with c-myc, a oncogene product, and inhibit apoptosis (Shichiri et al., 1999). It has been also reported that the v-Myc oncoprotein represses AM gene expression in mouse fibroblasts, and they attributed this Myc-mediated repression to the initiator element (INR) in the promoter region of the mouse AM gene (Wang et al., 1999). Although the consensus sequence for INR does not exist in the promoter region of the human AM gene, it has been shown that AM exerts a wide range of effects on cell growth and apoptosis. On the one hand AM has been shown to promote growth and suppress apoptosis of vascular endothelial cells (Miyashita et al., 2003; Kato et al., 1997, on the other hand it has been reported that AM inhibits proliferation and facilitates apoptosis of glomerular mesangial cells (Osajima et al., 1999; Parameswaran et al., 1999). Therefore, the expression of the AM gene may have some relation to oncogenesis or carcinogenesis.
Based on the various findings on AM gene expression described above, Figure 4 shows the putative mechanism of transcriptional regulation of the AM gene.

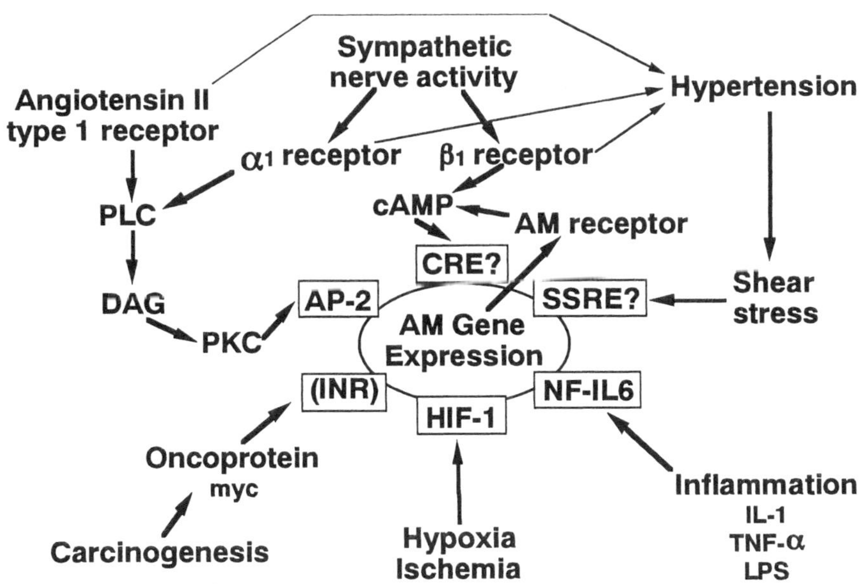

Figure 4. Putative regulatory mechanism of adrenomedullin (AM) gene expression. PLC,

phospholipase C; DAG, diacylglycerol; PKC, protein kinase C; IL-1, interleukin-1; TNF-α, tumor necrosis factor α; LPS, lipopolysaccharide; AP-2, activator protein 2; CRE, cAMP responsive element; SSRE, shear stress responsive element; NF-IL6, nuclear factor for interleukin-6 expression; HIF-1, hypoxia-inducible factor-1; INR, initiator element.

4. POLYMORPHISMS OF HUMAN AM GENE

(1) Microsatellite DNA Polymorphism of Human AM Gene

Nucleotide sequencing of genomic DNA adjacent to the human AM gene revealed that there is a microsatellite marker with a variable number of cytosine adenine (CA)-repeats at 4 kb downstream from the 3'-end of the AM gene (Figure 1) (Ishimitsu et al., 2001a). We investigated the relation of this microsatellite DNA polymorphism flanking to the 3'-end of AM gene with genetic predispositions to develop various cardiovascular diseases. Genomic DNA was extracted from peripheral leukocytes of 300 normal healthy subjects (NH), 143 patients with essential hypertension (EH), 111 patients with coronary artery disease (CAD), 128 hemodialysis patients with type 2 diabetes mellitus (DM-HD) and 106 type 2 diabetic patients without nephropathy (DM) (Ishimitsu et al., 2001b, Ishimitsu et al., 2003). The microsatellite region containing CA repeats was amplified by PCR using fluorescence labeled primers. An aliquot of the PCR product was electrophoresed on a urea-polyacrylamide gel and the number of CA-repeat was determined by measuring the length of amplified DNA fragment.

In the Japanese population, there existed four types of alleles with different CA-repeat numbers; 11, 13, 14 and 19. Figure 5 depicted the frequency of each allele in NH was 11: 28.8%, 13: 33.5%, 14: 34.7% and 19: 3.0%, respectively. As compared with this, the frequency of 19-CA-repeat allele was significantly increased to 7.3% in EH. The frequency of 19-repeat allele in CAD was 2.3% that was not significantly different from the frequency in NH. In DM-HD, the 19-repeat allele frequency was 9.0% and was higher than the frequency in NH, although the frequency of 19-repeat allele in DM without nephropathy was not significantly different from NH. The frequencies of 11-, 13- and 14-repeat alleles were not significantly different among NH, EH, CAD, DM and DM-HD.

These findings suggest that the 19-CA-repeat allele of microsatellite DNA polymorphism adjacent to the human AM gene is associated with the genetic predispositions to essential hypertension and diabetic nephropathy in Japanese subjects. However, this gene polymorphism is not likely to have association with predispositions to develop coronary artery diseases or type 2 diabetes mellitus itself.

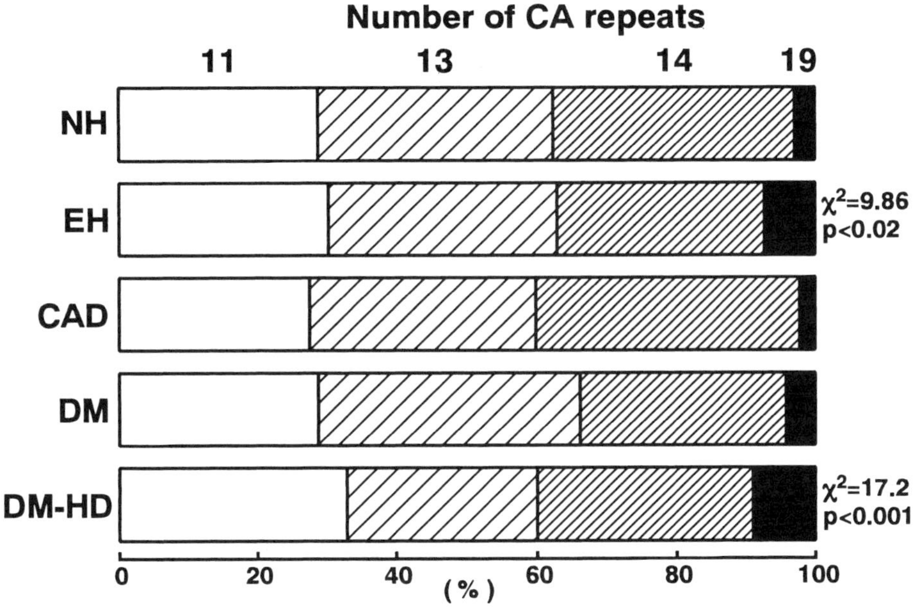

Figure 5. The frequency distribution of 11-, 13-, 14- and 19-CA-repeat alleles of the microsatellite polymorphism adjacent to the human AM gene in healthy subjects (NH), patients with essential hypertension (EH), patients with coronary artery disease (CAD), type 2 diabetic patients without nephropathy (DM) and hemodialysis patients with type 2 diabetes mellitus (DM HD).

(2) Single Nucleotide Polymorphism of Human AM Gene

In addition to the CA-repeat polymorphism downstream of the AM gene, there may exist some single nucleotide polymorphisms (SNP) in the human AM gene and the adjacent region. Numerous SNPs of this sort have already been recognized, and some of them are thought to confer a genetic predisposition to develop cardiovascular disorders (Daley et al., 2001). Therefore, it may be worthwhile to investigate such SNPs in the AM gene in relation to the gene function and predisposition to cardiovascular diseases.

Considering the prominent bioactivity of AM in the cardiovascular system, such SNPs of the AM gene may also have some relation to the pathophysiology of cardiovascular disorders.

In order to explore the variation of human AM gene, we amplified the 3180 bp genomic DNA encoding AM cDNA and its 5'-flanking region by PCR in 8 fragments. They were directly sequenced and the nucleotide sequence was compared in 24 subjects. Consequently, two single nucleotide polymorphisms were discovered in introns 1 and 3. In 3 of 24 subjects, +223A in intron 1 was replaced by C which creates the recognition site of restriction enzyme Mva I. In the same 3 subjects, +1100C in intron 3 was replaced by G. Therefore, these two SNPs are supposed to link each other.

The genotype of +223A/C polymorphism of AM gene was examined in 588 subjects who entered the health-check program of our hospital and did not have any diseases currently treated. The genomic DNA fragment containing this +223A/C was amplified by PCR, digested with Mva I, and then electrophoresed on agarose gel. The frequencies of AA, AC and CC genotypes were 92.5%, 7.5% and 0.0%, respectively. This SNP of AM gene may also have some relation to genetic predisposition or risk factors of cardiovascular diseases.

Thus far, a number of gene polymorphisms have been suggested to confer a predisposition to cardiovascular diseases (Danser et al., 2000; Tang et al., 2001; Carluccio et al., 2001). Most of them are related to genes of cardiovascular hormones and their signal transduction systems. Some of these gene polymorphisms have been shown to affect the expression of genes or the activity of gene products (Rigat et al., 1990; Jeunemaitre et al., 1992). Because the plasma AM levels are not different among the genotypes, the microsatellite CA-repeat polymorphism examined in our study is unlikely to affect expression of the AM gene (Ishimitsu et al., 2001b). It may be possible that this microsatellite polymorphism is associated with the function of other genes, because the number of short tandem repeats may affect the conformation of DNA and thereby may affect the transcription of nearby genes. In this context, it should be noted that several genes, such as shingomyelinase, parathyroid hormone, and lactate dehydrogenase, are known to be located near the AM gene in the short arm of chromosome 11.

Microsatellite markers, like the one we examined, consist of a variable number of repeats of short nucleotides, and hundreds of such repeat markers are thought to be scattered throughout the genomic DNA. These microsatellite markers can be utilized to locate the genomic region responsible for hereditary diseases or traits. Until now several diseases have been shown to be associated with such microsatellite DNA polymorphism. For example, the CA-repeat polymorphism lying upstream of the aldose reductase gene affects the development of nephropathy and retinopathy in type 1 diabetes mellitus (Heesom et al., 1997), and a certain number of TCAT repeats in intron 1 of the tyrosine hydroxylase gene has been associated with genetic predisposition to develop essential hypertension (Sharma P et al., 1998). Accumulation of information about the association of cardiovascular disorders with various microsatellite markers may serve to clarify the genetic risks of cardiovascular diseases that are attributed to multiple genomic regions.

CONCLUSION

Together, the accumulated results from experimental and clinical studies reveal that AM is involved in the defense of the cardiovascular endocrine system against the progression of organ injuries and dysfunction. Production of AM is increased in various cardiovascular disorders, such as hypertension, heart failure and renal failure (Ishimitsu et al., 1994a; Nishikimi et al., 1995; Kato et al., 1999; Kohno et al., 1996). AM dilates the blood vessels and improves regional blood flow. In addition, AM inhibits the growth and migration of vascular smooth muscle cells and thereby inhibits cardiovascular hypertrophy (Kano et al., 1996; Horio et al., 1995). AM exhibits a natriuretic effect in the kidneys and inhibits bronchoconstriction in the lungs. These versatile actions of AM are thought to help prevent the vicious cycle leading to cardiovascular organ failure. Thus, it is suggested that AM plays a significant role in the pathophysiology of the cardiovascular system. Future analyses of the structure and variation of the AM gene should further clarify the theoretical basis of AM gene function and its implication in the pathogenesis of cardiovascular diseases.

REFERENCES

Arnold A, Kim HG, Gaz RD, Eddy RL, Fukushima Y, Byers MG, Shows TB,

Kronenberg HM. (1989) Molecular cloning and chromosomal mapping of DNA rearranged with the parathyroid hormone gene in a parathyroid adenoma. J Clin Invest 83:2034-2040.

Autelitano DJ, Ridings R, Tang F. (2001) Adrenomedullin is a regulated modulator of neonatal cardiomyocyte hypertrophy in vitro. Cardiovasc Res 51:255-264.

Barker S, Wood E, Clark AJ, Corder R. (1998) Cloning of bovine preproadrenomedullin and inhibition of its basal expression in vascular endothelial cells by staurosporine. Life Sci 62:1407-1415.

Cameron VA, Autelitano DJ, Evans JJ, Ellmers LJ, Espiner EA, Nicholls MG, Richards AM. (2002) Adrenomedullin expression in rat uterus is correlated with plasma estradiol. Am J Physiol Endocrinol Metab 282:E139-E146.

Carluccio M, Soccio M, De Caterina R. (2001) Aspects of gene polymorphisms in cardiovascular disease: the renin-angiotensin system. Eur J Clin Invest 31:476-488.

Chun TH, Itoh H, Ogawa Y, Tamura N, Takaya K, Igaki T, Yamashita J, Doi K, Inoue M, Masatsugu K, Korenaga R, Ando J, Nakao K. (1997) Shear stress augments expression of C-type natriuretic peptide and adrenomedullin. Hypertension 29:1296-1302.

Chun TH, Itoh H, Saito T, Yamahara K, Doi K, Mori Y, Ogawa Y, Yamashita J, Tanaka T, Inoue M, Masatsugu K, Sawada N, Fukunaga Y, Nakao K. (2000) Oxidative stress augments secretion of endothelium-derived relaxing peptides, C-type natriuretic peptide and adrenomedullin. J Hypertens 18:575-580.

Cormier-Regard S, Nguyen SV, Claycomb WC. (1998) Adrenomedullin gene expression is developmentally regulated and induced by hypoxia in rat ventricular cardiac myocytes. J Biol Chem 273:17787-17792.

Daley GQ, Cargill M. (2001) The heart SNPs a beat: polymorphisms in candidate genes for cardiovascular disease. Trends Cardiovasc Med 11:60-66.

Danser AH, Schunkert H (2000) Renin-angiotensin system gene polymorphisms: potential mechanisms for their association with cardiovascular diseases. Eur J Pharmacol 410:303-316.

da Veiga Pereira L, Desnick RJ, Adler DA, Disteche CM, Schuchman EH. (1991) Regional assignment of the human acid sphingomyelinase gene (SMPD1) by PCR analysis of somatic cell hybrids and in situ hybridization to 11p15.1----p15.4. Genomics 9:229-234.

Dotsch J, Harmjanz A, Christiansen H, Hanze J, Lampert F, Rascher W. (2000)

Gene expression of neuronal nitric oxide synthase and adrenomedullin in human neuroblastoma using real-time PCR. Int J Cancer 88:172-175.
Giacalone PL, Vuaroqueaux V, Daures JP, Houafic L, Martin PM, Laffargue F, Maudelonde T. (2003) Expression of adrenomedullin in human ovaries, ovarian cysts and cancers. Correlation with estrogens receptor status. Eur J Obstet Gynecol Reprod Biol 110:224-229.
Hata K, Takebayashi Y, Akiba S, Fujiwaki R, Iida K, Nakayama K, Nakayama S, Fukumoto M, Miyazaki K. (2000) Expression of the adrenomedullin gene in epithelial ovarian cancer. Mol Hum Reprod 6:867-872.
Heesom AE, Hibberd ML, Millward A, Demaine AG. (1997) Polymorphism in the 5'-end of the aldose reductase gene is strongly associated with the development of diabetic nephropathy in type I diabetes. Diabetes 46:287-291.
Hirata Y, Mitaka C, Sato K, Nagura T, Tsunoda Y, Amaha K, Marumo F. (1996) Increased circulating adrenomedullin, a novel vasodilatory peptide, in sepsis. J Clin Endocrinol Metab 81:1449-1453.
Hofbauer KH, Schoof E, Kurtz A, Sandner P. (2002) Inflammatory cytokines stimulate adrenomedullin expression through nitric oxide-dependent and -independent pathways. Hypertension 39:161-167.
Horio T, Kohno M, Kano H, Ikeda M, Yasunari K, Yokokawa K, Minami M, Takeda T. (1995) Adrenomedullin as a novel antimigration factor of vascular smooth muscle cells. Circ Res 77:660-664.
Ishimitsu T, Nishikimi T, Saito Y, Kitamura K, Eto T, Kangawa K, Matsuo H, Omae T, Matsuoka H. (1994a) Plasma levels of adrenomedullin, a newly identified hypotensive peptide, in patients with hypertension and renal failure. J Clin Invest 94:2158-2161.
Ishimitsu T, Kojima M, Kangawa K, Hino J, Matsuoka H, Kitamura K, Eto T, Matsuo H. (1994b) Genomic structure of human adrenomedullin gene. Biochem Biophys Res Commun 203:631-639.
Ishimitsu T, Miyata A, Matsuoka H, Kangawa K. (1998) Transcriptional regulation of human adrenomedullin gene in vascular endothelial cells. Biochem Biophys Res Commun 243:463-470.
Ishimitsu T, Minami J, Nishikimi T, Yoshida K, Tsukada H, Kangawa K, Matsuoka H. (1999) Changes in plasma adrenomedullin in physiological and pathological conditions in human subjects. J Cardiovasc Pharmacol

34(Suppl 4):S47-S51.

Ishimitsu T, Hosoya K, Tsukada K, Minami J, Ono H, Ohrui M, Hino J, Kangawa K, Matsuoka H (2001a) Chromosomal sublocalization and microsatellite DNA polymorphism of human adrenomedullin gene. Peptides 22:1739-1744.

Ishimitsu T, Hosoya K, Tsukada K, Minami J, Futoh Y, Ono H, Ohrui M, Hino J, Kangawa K, Matsuoka H. (2001b) Microsatellite DNA polymorphism of human adrenomedullin gene in normotensive subjects and patients with essential hypertension. Hypertension 38:9-12.

Ishimitsu T, Tsukada K, Minami J, Ono H, Ohrui M, Hino J, Kangawa K, Matsuoka H. (2003) Microsatellite DNA polymorphism of human adrenomedullin gene in type 2 diabetic patients with renal failure. Kidney Int 63:2230-2235.

Isumi Y, Shoji H, Sugo S, Tochimoto T, Yoshioka M, Kangawa K, Matsuo H, Minamino N. (1998) Regulation of adrenomedullin production in rat endothelial cells. Endocrinology 139:838-846.

Jeunemaitre X, Soubrier F, Kotelevtsev YV, Lifton RP, Williams CS, Charru A, Hunt SC, Hopkins PN, Williams RR, Lalouel JM, Corvol P. (1992) Molecular basis of human hypertension: role of angiotensinogen. Cell 71:169-180.

Jimenez N, Abasolo I, Jongsma J, Calvo A, Garayoa M, van der Kwast TH, van Steenbrugge GJ, Montuenga LM. (2003) Androgen-independent expression of adrenomedullin and peptidylglycine alpha-amidating monooxygenase in human prostatic carcinoma. Mol Carcinog 38:14-24.

Jougasaki M, Grantham JA, Redfield MM, Burnett JC Jr. (2001) Regulation of cardiac adrenomedullin in heart failure. Peptides 22:1841-1850.

Kano H, Kohno M, Yasunari K, Yokokawa K, Horio T, Ikeda M, Minami M, Hanehira T, Takeda T, Yoshikawa J. (1996) Adrenomedullin as a novel antiproliferative factor of vascular smooth muscle cells. J Hypertens 14:209-213.

Kapas S, Tenchini ML, Farthing PM. (2001) Regulation of adrenomedullin secretion in cultured human skin and oral keratinocytes. J Invest Dermatol 117:353-359.

Kato H, Shichiri M, Marumo F, Hirata Y. (1997) Adrenomedullin as an autocrine/paracrine apoptosis survival factor for rat endothelial cells. Endocrinology 138:2615-2620.

Kato J, Kitamura K, Matsui E, Tanaka M, Ishizaka Y, Kita T, Kangawa K, Eto T.

(1999) Plasma adrenomedullin and natriuretic peptides in patients with essential or malignant hypertension. Hypertens Res 22:61-65.

Katsuki A, Sumida Y, Gabazza EC, Murashima S, Urakawa H, Morioka K, Kitagawa N, Tanaka T, Araki-Sasaki R, Hori Y, Nakatani K, Yano Y, Adachi Y. (2002) Acute hyperinsulinemia is associated with increased circulating levels of adrenomedullin in patients with type 2 diabetes mellitus. Eur J Endocrinol 147:71-75.

Kitamura K, Kangawa K, Kawamoto M, Ichiki Y, Nakamura S, Matsuo H, Eto T: (1993a) Adrenomedullin: a novel hypotensive peptide isolated from human pheochromocytoma. Biochem Biophys Res Commun 192:553-560.

Kitamura K, Sakata J, Kangawa K, Kojima M, Matsuo H, Eto T: (1993b) Cloning and characterization of cDNA encoding a precursor for human adrenomedullin. Biochem Biophys Res Commun 194:720-725.

Kitamura K, Ichiki Y, Tanaka M, Kawamoto M, Emura J, Sakakibara S, Kangawa K, Matsuo H, Eto T: (1994) Immunoreactive adrenomedullin in human plasma. FEBS Lett 341:288-290.

Kobayashi H, Yamamoto R, Kitamura K, Niina H, Masumoto K, Minami SI, Yanagita T, Izumi F, Aunis D, Eto T, Wada A. (1999) Cyclic AMP-dependent synthesis and release of adrenomedullin and proadrenomedullin N-terminal 20 peptide in cultured bovine adrenal chromaffin cells. Eur J Biochem 263:702-708.

Kohno M, Hanehira T, Kano H, Horio T, Yokokawa K, Ikeda M, Minami M, Yasunari K, Yoshikawa J. (1996) Plasma adrenomedullin concentrations in essential hypertension. Hypertension 27:102-107.

Ladoux A, Frelin C. (2000) Coordinated Up-regulation by hypoxia of adrenomedullin and one of its putative receptors (RDC-1) in cells of the rat blood-brain barrier. J Biol Chem 275:39914-39919.

Letizia C, Subioli S, Cerci S, Caliumi C, Verrelli C, Delfini E, Celi M, Scuro L, D' Erasmo E. (2002) High plasma adrenomedullin concentrations in patients with high-renin essential hypertension. J Renin Angiotensin Aldosterone Syst 3:126-129.

Letizia C, Caliumi C, Delfini E, Celi M, Subioli S, Diacinti D, Minisola S, D'erasmo E, Mazzuoli GF. (2003) Adrenomedullin concentrations are elevated in plasma of patients with primary hyperparathyroidism.

Metabolism 52:159-162.

Li SS, Luedemann M, Sharief FS, Takano T, Deaven LL. (1988) Mapping of human lactate dehydrogenase-A, -B, and -C genes and their related sequences: the gene for LDHC is located with that for LDHA on chromosome 11. Cytogenet Cell Genet 48:16-18.

Luodonpaa M, Rysa J, Pikkarainen S, Tenhunen O, Tokola H, Puhakka J, Marttila M, Vuolteenaho O, Ruskoaho H. (2003) Mechanisms regulating adrenomedullin gene expression in the left ventricle: role of mechanical load. Regul Pept 112:153-159.

Miyashita K, Itoh H, Sawada N, Fukunaga Y, Sone M, Yamahara K, Yurugi T, Nakao K. (2003) Adrenomedullin promotes proliferation and migration of cultured endothelial cells. Hypertens Res 26 Suppl:S93-S98.

Nakayama M, Takahashi K, Kitamuro T, Murakami O, Shirato K, Shibahara S (2000) Transcriptional control of adrenomedullin induction by phorbol ester in human monocytic leukemia cells. Eur J Biochem 267:3559-3566.

Nishikimi T, Saito Y, Kitamura K, Ishimitsu T, Eto T, Kangawa K, Matsuo H, Omae T, Matsuoka H. (1995) Increased plasma levels of adrenomedullin in patients with heart failure. J Am Coll Cardiol 26:1424-1431.

Ogita T, Hashimoto E, Yamasaki M, Nakaoka T, Matsuoka R, Kira Y, Fujita T. (2001) Hypoxic induction of adrenomedullin in cultured human umbilical vein endothelial cells. J Hypertens 19:603-608.

Osajima A, Kato H, Uezono Y, Suda T, Okazaki M, Oishi Y, Tamura M, Tanaka H, Izumi F, Nakashima Y. (1999) Adrenomedullin inhibits transmural pressure induced mesangial cell proliferation through activation of protein kinase A. Nephron. 83:352-357.

Parameswaran N, Nambi P, Brooks DP, Spielman WS. (1999) Regulation of glomerular mesangial cell proliferation in culture by adrenomedullin. (1999) Eur J Pharmacol 372:85-95.

Rigat B, Hubert C, Alhenc-Gelas F, Cambien F, Corvol P, Soubrier F. (1990) An insertion/deletion polymorphism in the angiotensin I-converting enzyme gene accounting for half the variance of serum enzyme levels. J Clin Invest 86:1343-1346.

Rocchi P, Boudouresque F, Zamora AJ, Muracciole X, Lechevallier E, Martin PM, Ouafik L. (2001) Expression of adrenomedullin and peptide amidation activity in human prostate cancer and in human prostate cancer cell lines. Cancer Res 61:1196-1206.

Romppanen H, Marttila M, Magga J, Vuolteenaho O, Kinnunen P, Szokodi I,

Ruskoaho H (1997) Adrenomedullin gene expression in the rat heart is stimulated by acute pressure overload: blunted effect in experimental hypertension. Endocrinology 138:2636-2639.

Sharma P, Hingorani A, Jia H. Ashby M, Hopper R, Clayton D, Brown MJ. (1998) Positive association of tyrosine hydroxylase microsatellite marker to essential hypertension. Hypertension 32:676-682.

Shichiri M, Kato H, Doi M, Marumo F, Hirata Y. (1999) Induction of max by adrenomedullin and calcitonin gene-related peptide antagonizes endothelial apoptosis. Mol Endocrinol 13:1353-1363.

Shinoki N, Kawasaki T, Minamino N, Okahara K, Ogawa A, Ariyoshi H, Sakon M, Kambayashi J, Kangawa K, Monden M. (1998) Shear stress down-regulates gene transcription and production of adrenomedullin in human aortic endothelial cells. J Cell Biochem 71:109-115.

Sugo S, Minamino N, Kangawa K, Miyamoto K, Kitamura K, Sakata J, Eto T, Matsuo H. (1994a) Endothelial cells actively synthesize and secrete adrenomedullin. Biochem Biophys Res Commun 201:1160-1166.

Sugo S, Minamino N, Shoji H, Kangawa K, Kitamura K, Eto T, Matsuo H. (1994b) Production and secretion of adrenomedullin from vascular smooth muscle cells: augmented production by tumor necrosis factor-alpha. Biochem Biophys Res Commun 203:719-726.

Sugo S, Minamino N, Shoji H, Kangawa K, Matsuo H. (1995) Effects of vasoactive substances and cAMP related compounds on adrenomedullin production in cultured vascular smooth muscle cells. FEBS Lett 369:311-314.

Takahashi K, Udono-Fujimori R, Totsune K, Murakami O, Shibahara S. (2003) Suppression of cytokine-induced expression of adrenomedullin and endothelin-1 by dexamethasone in T98G human glioblastoma cells. Peptides. 24:1053-1062.

Tanaka T, Akiyama H, Kanai H, Sato M, Takeda S, Sekiguchi K, Yokoyama T, Kurabayashi M. (2002) Endothelial PAS domain protein 1 (EPAS1) induces adrenomedullin gene expression in cardiac myocytes: role of EPAS1 in an inflammatory response in cardiac myocytes. J Mol Cell Cardiol 34:739-748.

Tang Z, Tracy RP. (2001) Candidate genes and confirmed genetic polymorphisms associated with cardiovascular diseases: a tabular assessment. J Thromb

Thrombolys 11:49-81.

Tomoda Y, Kikumoto K, Isumi Y, Katafuchi T, Tanaka A, Kangawa K, Dohi K, Minamino N. (2001) Cardiac fibroblasts are major production and target cells of adrenomedullin in the heart in vitro. Cardiovasc Res 49:721-730.

Tsuruda T, Kato J, Kitamura K, Imamura T, Koiwaya Y, Kangawa K, Komuro I, Yazaki Y, Eto T. (2000) Enhanced adrenomedullin production by mechanical stretching in cultured rat cardiomyocytes. Hypertension 35:1210-1214.

Tsuruda T, Kato J, Kitamura K, Mishima K, Imamura T, Koiwaya Y, Kangawa K, Eto T. (2001) Roles of protein kinase C and Ca2+-dependent signaling in angiotensin II-induced adrenomedullin production in rat cardiac myocytes. J Hypertens 19:757-763.

Udono T, Totsune K, Takahashi K, Abe T, Sato M, Shibahara S, Tamai M. (2000) Increased expression of adrenomedullin mRNA in the tissues of intraocular and orbital tumors. Am J Ophthalmol 129:555-556.

Uemura T, Kato J, Kuwasako K, Kitamura K, Kangawa K, Eto T. (2002) Aldosterone augments adrenomedullin production without stimulating pro-adrenomedullin N-terminal 20 peptide secretion in vascular smooth muscle cells. J Hypertens 20:1209-1214.

Wang X, Yue TL, Barone FC, White RF, Clark RK, Willette RN, Sulpizio AC, Aiyar NV, Ruffolo RR Jr, Feuerstein GZ. (1995) Discovery of adrenomedullin in rat ischemic cortex and evidence for its role in exacerbating focal brain ischemic damage. Proc Natl Acad Sci U S A 92:11480-11484.

Wang X, Peters MA, Utama FE, Wang Y, Taparowsky EJ. (1999) The Adrenomedullin gene is a target for negative regulation by the Myc transcription complex. Mol Endocrinol 13:254-267.

4

ADRENOMEDULLIN EXPRESSION AND SECRETION

Naoto Minamino

National Cardiovascular Center Research Institute, Osaka, Japan

INTRODUCTION

Adrenomedullin (AM) is a 52-residue vasodilatory peptide originally isolated from extracts of human pheochromocytoma tissue (Kitamura, 1993a; Kitamura, 1993b). This peptide was first deduced to be expressed and secreted from adrenal medulla, and to regulate the cardiovascular system as a hormone. AM was actually detected in the plasma, and its concentrations were elevated in patients with hypertension and other cardiovascular diseases (Eto, 1999). In the survey for AM-producing tissues and cells, however, low levels of immunoreactive (IR) AM were widely observed in addition to adrenal gland, heart and lung (Kitamura, 2002). We demonstrated the active expression and secretion of AM from vascular smooth muscle cells (VSMCs) and endothelial cells (ECs) (Sugo, 1994a, b). By subsequent studies, AM was found to be secreted from cardiomyocytes, epithelial cells and fibroblasts, and every cell is now recognized to have an ability to express and secrete AM (Isumi, 1998a; Tomoda, 200b; Minamino 2002). In the cases of classical peptide hormones, endocrine cells synthesize and store the peptides in the granules, and secrete them in response to stimulation through the regulated pathway. In the non-endocrine cells, such as VSMCs, peptides are constitutively secreted soon after synthesis. As a result, the tissue concentration of AM is often dissociated from its mRNA level depending on the secretion pathway of constituent cells. In this review, therefore, regulation of AM expression and secretion is described based on the secretion rates from cultured cells, which I hope helps elucidate the physiological function of AM.

1. AM EXPRESSION AND SECRETION IN VARIOUS CELLS

(1) Vascular Endothelial Cells and Smooth Muscle Cells

Next to adrenal chromaffin cells, ECs and VSMCs were verified to actively secrete AM. The secretion rate of AM from rat EC and VSMC was parallel to the synthesis of AM, and correlated with AM mRNA level (Sugo, 1995; Isumi, 1998b), as AM is expressed, synthesized and secreted constitutively from EC and VSMC.
The secretion rates of AM from aortic ECs (AECs) of rat, human, bovine and porcine origin were measured to be 1.83, 1.55, 0.38, 2.02 fmol/10^5 cells/h, respectively (Sugo, 1994a; Tomoda, 2001b). Human umbilical vein EC (HUVEC), bovine aortic and carotid artery ECs, and canine aortic EC secreted AM at rates of 0.54, 0.91, and 0.39 fmol/10^5 cells/h, respectively (Udono, 2001; Michibata, 1998; Chun, 2000). Secretion rates of AM from rat, human, bovine, and porcine aortic smooth muscle cells (ASMC) were 0.43, 1.77, 0.57, and 0.91,respectively (Sugo, 1994b; Tomoda, 2001b). AM gene expression was observed in cultured rat AEC and ASMC (Sugo, 1994a, b; Isumi, 1998b). At the tissue level, AM and/or AM mRNA were detected in canine ASMC, porcine AEC and VSMC of the aorta, pulmonary artery, pulmonary vein, renal artery and coronary artery, human lung EC and VSMC (Jougasaki, 1995; Martinez, 1995; Nishimura, 1997). Taken together, AM is synthesized and secreted from ECs and VSMCs including arteries and veins at relatively comparable rates.
Regulation profiles of AM secretion from rat EC and VSMC are summarized in Table 1. In this review, up- and down-regulation of AM expression and secretion are indicated by the direction of arrows, and the degree of alteration in the AM secretion is indicated by the number of arrows. Interleulkin 1 showed stimulatory effects on AM secretion from rat AEC, and tumor necrosis factor (TNF) and lipopolysaccharide (LPS) also augmented it. Instead, transforming growth factor β_1 (TGF-β_1) and interferon γ (IFN-γ) inhibited AM secretion. Glucocorticoid and thyroid hormone (T_3) were common stimulators of AM secretion from ECs, and aldosterone and sex steroids also increased it. Thrombin induced a strong effect, but the

direction of its effect was different in each EC. In most cases, AM secretion rates correlated with AM gene expression levels in rat AECs. Based on these results, TNF-α, LPS, IL-1β, glucocorticoid and T_3 are the stimulators of AM expression and secretion from the ECs.

In the case of VSMCs, more uniform regulation of AM secretion was observed. Pro-inflammatory cytokines (IL-1 and TNF) and LPS increased the AM secretion rate from VSMCs, while IFN-γ suppressed it. Glucocorticoids, mineralocoroticoid and T_3 increased the AM secretion rate, which was compatible with AM mRNA levels.

In ECs and VSMCs, pro-inflammatory cytokines, LPS, steroid and thyroid hormones, IFN-γ and TGF-β_1 are common stimulators or suppressors. Basic FGF and EGF suppressed AM secretion from EC but elevated it from VSMC. IL-2, adrenaline, noradrenaline and peptide hormones altered AM secretion rate, but did not induced the same effect on EC and VSMC. Forskolin, an adenylyl cyclase stimulator, increased AM secretion rate from VSMC, and phorbol ester, a protein kinase C stimulator, elevated AM secretion rate from both cells in a low concentration but decreased in a high concentration. Fetal calf serum (FCS) stimulated AM secretion from VSMC but suppressed it from EC. These data clarified that many substances participate in the regulation of AM secretion from vascular wall cells in rather complex manners.

Oxygen concentration and physical stress alter AM secretion from EC and VSMC. Hypoxia is a potent stimulus of AM expression and secretion, and highly elevated levels of AM mRNA were observed in the ECs and VSMCs of both cell culture and tissue (Nakayama, 1999a). As for the shear stress, different results were obtained for human AEC and HUVEC (Chun, 1997; Shinoki, 1998). As Marutsuka *et al.* (2003) observed the higher IR-AM at the branching portions and in the inner aspect of the curvature of the aortic arch, AM synthesis is considered to be elevated *in vivo* under the high shear stress conditions.

AM secretion rates are not so uniform even in the ECs or VSMCs prepared from the same tissue (Tomoda, 2001b), but the regulation

Table 1. Effects of various substances on AM secretion from aortic EC, SMC and fibroblasts.

Substance	Rat AEC	Rat ASMC	Mouse 3T3	Human NHLF
IL-1α	↑↑	↑↑↑(↑)		
IL-1β	↑	↑↑↑(↑)	↑	↑
IL-2	—	↑		
TNF-α	↑↑(↑)	↑↑↑(↑)	↑↑	↑
TNF-β	↑	↑↑↑(↑)		
LPS	↑	↑↑↑(↑)	↑	—
TGF-β_1	↓↓(↓)	—	↓↓↓	↓↓↓
basic FGF	↓	↑	↑	↓
EGF	↓	↑	—	↓
IFN-γ	↓	↓	↓↓	↓
Hydrocortisone	↑	↑↑(↑)		
Dexamethasone	↑(↑)	↑↑(↑)	↑↑	↑
Aldosterone	↑	↑↑		
Testosterone	↑	—		
Progesterone	↑	↑		
17β-estradiol	↑	—		
T_3	↑(↑)	↑(↑)	↑	—
Adrenaline	—	↑		
Noradrenaline	↑	—		
VIP	—	↓		
CGRP	↓	—		
Endothelin-1	↓	↑		
Angiotensin II	—	↑		
Substance P	—	↑		
Thrombin	↑↑(—)	↓↓↓(↓)	↑	↓↓↓
Phorbol ester	↑	↑		
Forskolin	—	↓↓↓(↓)	↓↓	—
Fetal calf serum	↓↓	↑		—
Hypoxia		↑(↑)		

—, Not significant; ↑, increase to101-200%; ↑↑, to 201-300%; ↑↑↑, to ≥ 300%; ↓, decrease to 67-99%; ↓↓, to 34-66%; ↓↓↓, to ≤ 33%. ( ) indicates data for AM mRNA; (↑), increase; (↓), decrease; (—), not significant. 3T3, embryonic fibroblast; NHLF, normal human lung fibroblast.

profiles are similar to each other. AM secreted from EC and VSMC is, therefore, deduced to elicit the definite effects for responding to the physiological conditions, such as inflammation and sepsis.
Aldosterone is recently shown to be synthesized in the vascular wall, and increases AM secretion level 2-3 fold (Eto, 2003). Like aldosterone or endothelin-1, many stimulants in Table 1 are secreted from the vascular wall, which in turn regulate AM expression and secretion. Thus, more efficient regulation of AM concentration is initiated when physiological stimuli are applied to the vasculature.

(2) Fibroblasts

Regulation of AM secretion from Swiss 3T3 embryonic fibroblast and normal human lung fibroblast (NHLF) is shown in Table 1, and their basal secretion rates of AM were 0.24 and 6.83 fmol/10^5 cells/h, respectively (Isumi, 1998a). Hs68 human skin fibroblast also secreted AM at a rate of 6.58 fmol/10^5 cells/h (Isumi, 1998a). Although only Swiss 3T3 cell shows a low secretion rate, the fibroblast is one of the cell groups that can secrete AM at a high rate contrary to our previous knowledge.
AM secretion from the fibroblasts is regulated by the profile similar to that of VSMCs (Isumi, 1998a). TNF-α, IL-1β and LPS were stimulators of AM secretion from the 3 fibroblasts although LPS did not alter it from NHLF. Dexamethasone stimulated, but TGF-β_1 and IFN-γ suppressed AM secretion. The effects of basic FGF and thrombin were opposite in the 2 fibroblasts shown in Table 1, and EGF, T_3 and forskolin did not induce the same effects. The similar regulation profiles of AM secretion from the fibroblast and VSMC indicate that the secreted AM from these 2 cell groups elicits similar effects especially in the inflammation.
In the case of patients with systemic inflammatory response syndrome (SIRS), including septic shock, plasma AM concentration was highly elevated (Hirata, 1996; Nishio, 1997; Ueda, 1999). In the LPS-injected rats, augmented AM gene expression was observed in almost all tissues, including liver and skeletal muscle (Shoji, 1995). These data suggest that the cells commonly present in all tissues are

sources of AM in the SIRS, and the fibroblasts and vascular wall cells are deduced to be major sources of AM.

(3) Cardiac Cells

Both rat cardiac myocyte and fibroblast actively secrete AM. AM secretion rate from neonatal cardiac myocyte was determined by 3 groups to be 0.92, 0.96 and 0.40 fmol/10^5 cells/h, while that from neonatal cardiac fibroblast to be 2.57, 0.51 and 0.50 fmol/10^5 cells/h (Tomoda, 2001a; Horio, 1998; Tsuruda, 1998, 1999). The regulation profile of AM secretion from cardiac fibroblast is the typical one of the fibroblast, and angiotensin II and endothelin-1 increased AM secretion rates about 1.5 fold (Tsuruda, 1999).

Table 2. Effects of various substances on AM secretion from rat cardiac myocyte and fibroblast.

Substance	Myocyte	Fibroblast
TNF-α	—	↑, ↑↑↑(↑)
IL-1β	—, ↑(↑)	↑↑, ↑↑↑(↑)
LPS	—	↑
TGF-β_1	—	↓↓
Dexamethasone	↑, ↑↑↑(↑)	↑↑
Angiotensin II	↑↑	↑
Endothelin-1	↑	↑
Fetal calf serum	↑↑↑	
Hypoxia (1%)	(↑)	
Stretch	↑(↑)	

Arrows and other symbols are the same as those used in Table 1.

Although inflammatory stimuli did not increase AM secretion from the cardiomyocyte, dexamethasone and FCS elicited strong effects on it (Tomoda, 2001a, Tsuruda,1999). Two types of cells present in the heart tissue have distinct profiles even in the AM expression and secretion, and the AM secreted from these cells is thought to exert different effects. In the tissue level, AM-positive immunostaining

was found in canine and human cardiomyocyte, rat cardiomyocyte, interstitium and EC (Jougasaki, 1995; Marutsuka, 2003).
Hypoxia increased AM expression in the cardiomyocyte (Cormier-Regard, 1998). Another feature in the case of cardiac cells is stretch-induced AM expression and secretion, which is observed only in the cardiomyocyte (Tsuruda, 1999). Both stretch- and angiotensin II-induced AM expression was inhibited with AT1 angiotensin II receptor antagonist (Eto, 2003). In the *in vivo* experiments, pressure overload induces left ventricular hypertrophy and up-regulates AM and atrial natriuretic peptide (ANP) expression. This induction is amplified with angiotensin II that is also synthesized at a high rate in the hypertrophic heart tissue. Monoclonal antibody against AM increases hypertrophic reaction and stimulates ANP synthesis and secretion (Tsuruda, 1998). Taken together, in the overloaded heart tissue, AM secretion is augmented by the stimulation of stretch and angiotensin II, and AM is expected to suppress the hypertrophy as a local mediator (Nishikimi, 2003).

(4) Epithelial Cells

AM was first detected in the bronchial epithelial cell (BE) (Martinez, 1995), and its secretion rate from human BE was 4.07 fmol/10^5 cells/h (Tomoda, 2001b). AM secretion rate was increased with TNF-α and suppressed by thrombin, but was not altered by other substances (Table 3). LLC-PK_1 porcine renal tubular epithelial cell secreted AM at a rate about 1/50 that of BE, but its regulation profile was similar to that of BE (Tomoda, 2001b). ARPE-19 human retinal pigment epithelial cells secreted AM at a rate of 3.14 fmol/10^5 cells/h, which was enhanced with IL-1β, IFN-γ and basic FGF. Hypoxia also augmented it from ARPE-19 (Udono, 2001).
Epithelial cells in trachea, urinary bladder and prostate, mammary gland, gallbladder as well as mucosal and glandular epithelial cells of the gastrointestinal tract were shown to express AM gene or synthesize AM by the RT-PCR, *in situ* hybridization and immunohistochemical method (Nishimura, 1997, Pewitt, 1999; Marutsuka, 2003). Calf BE expresses AM, but *in vivo* administration

of LPS did not alter the AM-immunostaining intensity as deduced. The epithelial cell is one of the major sources of AM, and the secreted AM acts as an exocrine factor in addition to an autocrine/paracrine factor. The regulation profile of AM secretion from the epithelial cell is not so highly regulated by the inflammation-related substances, indicating that its physiological effect is different from that of VSMC.

Table 3. Effects of various substances on AM secretion from epithelial cells.

Substance	Human BE	Pig LLC-PK$_1$	Human ARPE-19
TNF-α	↑	↑	—(—)
IL-1β	—	—	↑ (↑)
LPS	—	—	
IFN-γ	—	—	↑↑↑ (↑)
TGF-β$_1$		—	
Dexamethasone	—	—	
T$_3$		—	
Thrombin	↓↓	↓↓↓	
Forskolin	—		
Basic FGF			↑ (—)
Retinoic acid			—(—)
Hypoxia			↑(↑)

Arrows and other symbols are the same as those used in Table 1. BE, bronchial epithelial cell, LLC-PK$_1$, kidney epithelial cell; ARPE-1, retinal pigmental epithelial cell.

(5) Keratinocytes

Kapas *et al.* (2001) reported active synthesis of AM in human oral and skin keratinocytes (KCs), and their secretion rates were 2.12 and 2.93 fmol/10^5 cells/h, respectively (Table 3). AM secretion from oral KC was regulated in a manner similar to that of VSMC, except steroid hormones that had no effect on it. In contrast, AM secretion from skin KC was not stimulated with pro-inflammatory cytokines and LPS, but steroid hormones augmented it. TGF-β$_1$ and IFN-γ reduced AM secretion rate from both cells, and thrombin, phorbol ester, forskolin and dibutyryl-cAMP induced comparable effects on both cells in a manner similar to that of VSMC. Endothelin-1 enhanced and adrenocroticotropin (ACTH) lowered AM secretion from both KCs. Locally secreted AM is considered to be utilized as an autocrine/paracrine and exocrine factor, and AM secreted from the skin KC may have a role in the situations other than inflammation.

Table 4. Effects of various substances on AM secretion from keratinocytes and monocyte/macrophage.

Substance	Oral KC	Skin KC	RAW264.7	HL-60
IL-1α	↑	—		
IL-1β	↑	—	—	—
TNF-α	↑(↑)	—(—)	—	↑↑↑
TNF-β	↑	—		
LPS	↑(↑)	—(—)	↑↑↑(↑)	↑↑
TGF-β_1	↓(↓)	↓(↓)	↓	—
IFN-γ	↓	↓	↑↑↑	—
Hydrocortisone	—	↑	↓↓	
Dexamethasone	—	↑	↓↓↓	—
Aldosterone	—	↑		
Testosterone	—	↑		
Progesterone	—	↑		
Estradiol	—	↑	↓	
Endothelin-1	↑(↑)	↑(↑)		
ACTH	↓(↓)	↓(↓)		
Thrombin	↑	↑		
Phorbol ester	↑(—)	↑(↑)	↑	↑↑↑
Retinoic acid			↑	—
Forskolin	↓	↓	—	
Dibutyryl-cAMP	↓	—	—	
LDL			↑	
Acetyl LDL			↑	
Oxidized LDL			↑	

Arrows and other symbols are the same as those used in Table 1. Oral KC, human oral keratinocytes; Skin KC, human skin keratinocytes; RAW264.7, mouse peritoneal macrophage-derived cell; and HL-60, human promyelocytic leukemia cell.

(6) Blood Cells

AM synthesis and secretion was confirmed in the human peripheral blood granulocyte, lymphocyte, monocyte, monocyte-derived macrophage and mouse peritoneal macrophage, and their secretion rates were 2.95, 3.95, 8.50, 38.3, 8.33 amol/10^5 cells/h, respectively (Kubo, 1998a, b). AM secretion was observed in the monocyte- and macrophage-derived cell lines, but their secretion rates are also much lower than that of VSMC (Kubo, 1998a, b). AM gene expression and synthesis was observed in human lung alveolar macrophage, and its secretion rate was 37.1 amol/10^5 cells/h (Nakayama, 1999b).
From the regulation profiles of AM secretion from RAW264.7 and HL-60 (Table 4), LPS is deduced to be a common stimulator of AM secretion in the monocyte/macrophage family, and TNF-α and IL-1β showed weak effects on these cells. In the case of undifferentiated cells such as HL-60, AM secretion was stimulated with phorbol ester and/or retinoic acid, and its secretion rate was increased according to the degree of differentiation into macrophages (Kubo, 1998a). Glucocorticoids that inhibit the differentiation suppressed AM secretion from RAW264.7 cell (Kubo, 1998b). Thus, the differentiation into macrophage is found to induce AM expression. IFN-γ as well as low density lipoprotein (LDL) and its derivatives elevated AM secretion rate from RAW264.7 cell. This regulation profile is similar to that of TNF-α, IL-1β and inducible nitric oxide synthase, indicating that AM expression from the monocyte/macrophage is regulated by the mechanism similar to that of inflammation-related proteins.

(7) Adipocytes

Adipose tissue is now recognized as an endocrine tissue secreting a series of hormones and regulators such as leptin, adiponectin and TNF-α (Matsuzawa, 2004). NIH 3T3-L1 cells were often used as an adipocyte model, and confluent NIH 3T3 cells (non-adipocytes) were differentiated into adipocytes by the definite stimulation. AM secretion rates from pre-adipocyte and adipocyte were 3.77 and 1.51

fmol/10^5 cells/h, respectively (Li, 2003). TNF-α increased it more than 3-fold in both cells. IL-1β only enhanced AM secretion in pre-adipocyte, and IFN-γ did not alter it either cell (Table 5). The relatively high level of AM secretion from this adipocyte model suggests that AM is expressed and secreted from the adipose tissue, although differentiation into the adipocyte reduces the AM secretion rate and responses to the stimulation.

Table 5. Effects of inflammatory cytokines on AM secretion from adipocyte and astrocyte.

Substance	Mouse 3T3-L1 adipocyte	Mouse 3T3-L1 preadipocyte	Human normal astrocyte
TNF-α	↑↑↑(↑)	↑↑↑(↑)	↑↑↑(—)
IL-1β	—(—)	↑(↑)	↑↑↑(↑)
IFN-γ	—(—)	—(—)	↑↑↑(↑)

Arrows and other symbols are the same as those used in Table 1.

(8) Neurons, Glia, and Related Cells

In the histochemical analysis, AM-immunoreactive neurons are widely observed in the central nervous system (CNS), especially in the magnocellular system. At the cultured cell level, only AM secretion rate from PC12 cell was measured to be 0.155 fmol/10^5 cells/h (Tomoda, 2001b). TNF-α and dexamethasone stimulated AM secretion from PC12 cell, although IL-1β, LPS and IFN-γ did note alter it (Table 6).

Human brain astrocyte secreted AM at a rate of 1.17 fmol/10^5 cells/h, which was augmented more than 20 fold with IFN-γ, TNF-α and IL-1β (Takahashi, 2000a). C6 glioma cell secreted AM at a rate of 0.93 fmol/10^5 cells/h, and its regulation profile of AM secretion was rather different (Table 6). TGF-β_1, dexamethasone, T_3 and forskolin increased AM secretion, while TNF-α and IL-1β suppressed it. AM secretion rate from glioblastoma T98G cell was high (8.56 fmol/10^5 cells/h), which was elevated with IFN-γ and IL-1β but not with TNF-α(Takahashi, 1997). In the rat astrocyte stimulated with IFN-γ, AM mRNA was identified as one of the highly inducible genes by the differential display method. Thus, IFN-γ is a stimulator on AM secretion from glia and its tumor cells. Active secretion of AM from the glia cell in the CNS reminds us of that from the mesenchymal fibroblast in the peripheral tissue.

Table 6. Effects of various substances on AM secretion from tumor-derived cells.

Substance	GH_3	C_6	T98G	PC12	SW-13	DLD-1
TNF-α	↑↑	↓	↓(↓)	↑	↑(↑)	
IL-1β	—	↓	↑(↑)	—	↑(—)	
LPS	—	—		—		
IFN-γ	↓	—	↑(↑)	—	—(—)	↑(↑)
TGF-β_1	↑	↑				
Dexamethasone—	↑↑↑		↑	—		
T_3	↑	↑		—		
Thrombin	—	—		—		
Forskolin	↑	↑		↓		
ACTH					—	
Angiotensin II					—	
Hypoxia			↑↑(↑)			↑↑↑(↑)
Cobalt chloride			↑↑↑(↑)			↑↑↑(↑)

Arrows and other symbols are the same as those used in Table 1. GH_3, rat pituitary tumor cell secreting prolactin and growth hormone; C_6, rat brain glioma cell; T98G, human glioblatstoma cell; PC12, rat pheochromocytoma cell; SW-13, human adrenocortical carcinoma cell; DLD-1, colorectal adenocarcinoma cell.

(9) Tumor Cells

AM expression was observed many tumor cell lines. A secretion rate of AM from GH_3 pituitary tumor cell was 0.055 fmol/10^5 cells/h (Tomoda, 2001b). TGF-β_1 and forskolin elicited opposite effects on AM secretion from GH_3 cell, and glucocorticoid and LPS did not alter it (Table 6). SW-13 adrenocortical carcinoma cell secreted AM at a rate of 1.15 fmol/10^5 cells/h (Takahashi, 2000b), and TNF-α and IL-1β stimulated AM secretion. In the primarily cultured Cushing's adenoma cell, ACTH, dibutyryl-cAMP, staurosporine and H7 were reported to suppress AM gene transcription, while phorbol ester augmented it (Kapas, 1998). DLD-1 colorectal adenocarcinoma cell secreted AM at a rate of 0.050 fmol/10^5 cells/h, and IFN-γ increased AM secretion 2 fold. It is difficult to deduce the common features of AM secretion from these data, but hypoxia and hypoxia mimetic potently induce AM expression and secretion from T98G and DLD-1 cells.

(10) Other AM-Secreting Cells

A secretion rate of AM from rat mesangial cell was reported to be 0.26 fmol/10^5 cells/h (Michibata, 1998), and TNF-α and IL-1β increased it 6.25 and 4.5 fold (Chini, 1997). Human mesangial cell also secreted AM, and its secretion and expression was augmented with TNF-α, FCS and 8-Br-cAMP (Lai, 1998). Three different renal tubular epithelial cells (LLC-PK$_1$, MDCK and MDBK) secreted AM at low rates of 0.013-0.083 fmol/10^5 cells/h, and [Arg^8]-vasopressin stimulated AM secretion (Sato, 1998). These data suggest specific effects of AM in the renal system.

Bovine adrenal chromaffin cell secreted AM at a rate of 0.68 fmol/10^5 cells/h, and dibutyryl-cAMP and cholinergic stimulation increased its secretion rate (Kobayashi, 1999).

Female reproductive tissue contains many types of cells expressing and secreting AM (Cameron, 1998; Marutsuka 2003), which is highly regulated with hormones. AM gene expression in rat ovary granulosa cell was suppressed with follicle-stimulating hormone and chorionic gonadotropin, indicating that AM secretion from the granulosa cell is reduced by the differentiation (Moriyama, 2000).

2. HYPOXIA AND OXIDATIVE STRESS

Hypoxia is one of the strongest stimuli of AM expression and secretion, which is a common feature of the regulation in most cell types. By the recent *in vivo* studies, many types of cells in the brain, kidney, lung, heart, adrenal gland, eye and other tissues are

shown to augment AM expression and synthesis after exposure to hypoxia (Sandner, 2004; Yin, 2004).
Hypoxia increased AM mRNA level 6.7-15.2 fold in rat brain microvessel EC, and 5.54 fold in human coronary artery EC after 12-15h exposure (Ladoux, 2000; Nakayama, 1999b). The response of VSMC to hypoxia was more moderate than EC (Nagata, 1999). AM expression and secretion from HUVEC was up-regulated under the hypoxic conditions and returned to the control level upon re-exposure to the normal oxygen environment. Primary culture rat astrocyte increased AM secretion 9.5 fold after 15h exposure to hypoxia, and mesangial cells, MDCK, PC12 and retinal pigmental cells also enhanced it (Ladoux, 2000; Nagata, 1999; Udono, 2001). Hypoxia stimulated AM gene expression in the rat adult cardiomyocyte (Cormier-Regard, 1998), and hypoxia and its mimetics stimulated AM expression and secretion from 11 tumor cell lines (Garayoa, 2000; Kitamuro, 2000).
As for the mechanism for AM expression by hypoxic stress, Garayoa *et al.* (2000) proposed that hypoxia-inducible factor-1 (HIF-1) mediated pathway is predominant, based on the data of cellular responses of HIF-1α and HIF-1β knockout mouse, effects of HIF-1 activity stimulators and inhibitors, and activation of gene expression through putative hypoxia response elements of AM gene. Hypoxic stimulation was also reported to stabilize AM mRNA, but more data supporting the HIF-1-mediated pathway have been accumulated for the hypoxia-induced AM expression (Makino, 2003; Leonard, 2003). Thyroid hormone, a stimulator of HIF-1 expression and synthesis, is another common inducer of AM expression and secretion (Ma, 2004). In the *in vivo* system, more efficient augmentation can be undertaken for AM expression under the hypoxic conditions.
Oxidative stress enhanced AM expression and secretion. Exposure of bovine EC to diluted hydrogen peroxide increased AM secretion rate 1.74 fold (Chun, 2000). In another model of oxidative stress, AM expression was also elevated in EC and VSMCs (Ando, 1998).
AM was reported to increase Bcl-2 and to inhibit hypoxic death of endometrial cancer cells. As a result, AM promotes tumor growth by rescuing necrotic cell death in the tumor tissue (Oehler, 2001). A

high level of AM secreted by the serious cell damage is expected to elicit anti-apoptotic and angiogenic activity, which provides favorable cytoprotective effects in the normal tissues but unfavorable propagation in the tumor tissue.

3. COMMON FEATURES OF AM EXPRESSION AND SECRETION

The important features for AM expression and secretion are i) AM is expressed and secreted from the cells lacking secretory granules, and ii) pro-inflammatory cytokines, LPS, and growth factors regulate AM secretion. Another important point is that serious or lethal stress to the cells, such as hypoxia, augments AM expression and secretion. In the case of the endocrine type cells, AM stored in the granules are secreted immediately after stimulation. On the other hand, it usually takes 1-2 h after stimulation to observe a significant increase of AM expression and secretion in the non-endocrine type cells. These facts suggest that AM is mainly designed to elicit its effects as a local mediator.

Based on the regulation profiles of AM secretion, cultured cells can be classified into at least 3 classes. Class I consists of fibroblasts, VSMCs, ECs and oral KC. In this class, TNF, IL-1, LPS and glucocorticoid typically stimulate AM gene expression and secretion, while TGF-β_1 and IFN-γ generally suppress them. Class II contains monocyte, macrophage and their related cells. The expression and secretion of AM from these cells are mainly regulated by the degree of differentiation into macrophage and by activation with LPS and inflammatory cytokines including IFN-γ. Class III is tentatively separated from Classes I and II. AM secreted from the different classes is deduced to have distinct targets and effects.

Oxygen and physical stresses are another important factors regulating AM gene expression and secretion. Among them, hypoxia is considered to be a strong and common stimulus. In the *in vivo* experiments, hypoxic, hemorrhagic and septic shock actually augmented gene expression of AM in many types of cells and tissues, and increased plasma AM concentration (Yoshibayashi, 1999; Ueda,

1999). Under the conditions that the cells are seriously damaged, such as inflammation and hypoxia, AM expression and secretion is confirmed to be dramatically enhanced both *in vitro* and *in vivo* systems.
AM is now known to elicit a wide range of biological activity including apoptosis-survival, angiogenic, anti-inflammatory and mitogenic/anti-mitogenic effects in addition to the vasodilatory effect (Kato 1997; Hague, 2000; Clementi 1999; Hinson, 2000). By the recent studies on AM-transgenic and knockout mice, mortality and tissue damage caused by endotoxin and oxidative stress are reported to be highly improved in the AM-overexpressing mice and to be exacerbated in the AM knockout mice (Shindo, 2000, Shimosawa, 2003; Niu, 2004). The regulation profile of AM expression and secretion as well as the ubiquitous expression of AM reveals that AM is not a classical peptide hormone but is a cytokine-like peptide regulating a wide range of cell function as a local mediator.

CONCLUSION

Although AM is classified into the CGRP superfamily, almost all cells can express and synthesize AM in contrast with CGRP that is mainly expressed in the neurons and thyroid gland. AM secretion is mainly regulated with inflammation-related substances, growth factors and hormones, but hypoxia and physical stresses are another important stimuli for AM expression and secretion. A series of biological effects of AM in the vasodilation, angiogenesis, proliferation and inflammation, along with AM expression in many types of cells indicate that AM can elicit its effects not only as a vasodilatory hormone but also as a local mediator for protecting cells and tissues.

REFERENCES

Ando K, Ito Y, Kumada M, and Fujita T. (1998) Oxidative stress increases adrenomedullin mRNA levels in cultured rat vascular smooth muscle cells. Hypertens Res 21:187-191.
Cameron VA, and Fleming AM. (1998) Novel sites of adrenomedullin gene

expression in mouse and rat tissues. Endocrinology 139:2253-2264.

Chini EN, Chini CC, Bolliger C, Jougasaki M, Grande JP, Burnett JC, and Dousa TP. (1997) Cytoprotective effects of adrenomedullin in glomerular cell injury: central role of cAMP signaling pathway. Kidney Int 52:917-925.

Chun TH, Itoh H, Ogawa Y, Tamura N, Takaya K, Igaki T, Yamashita J, Doi K, Inoue M, Masatsugu K, Korenaga R, Ando J, and Nakao K. (1997) Shear stress augments expression of C-type natriuretic peptide and adrenomedullin. Hypertension 29:1296-1302.

Chun TH, Itoh H, Saito T, Yamahara K, Doi K, Mori Y, Ogawa Y, Yamashita J, Tanaka T, Inoue M, Masatsugu K, Sawada N, Fukunaga Y, and Nakao K. (2000) Oxidative stress augments secretion of endothelium-derived relaxing peptides, C-type natriuretic peptide and adrenomedullin. J Hypertens 18:575-580.

Clementi G., Caruso A, Cutuli VM, Prato A, Mangano NG, and Amico Roxas M. (1999) Antiinflammatory activity of adrenomedullin in the acetic acid peritonitis in rats. Life Sci 65:P.L203-208.

Cormier-Regard S, Nguyen SV, and Claycomb WC. (1998) Adrenomedullin gene expression is developmentally regulated and induced by hypoxia in rat ventricular cardiac myocytes. J Biol Chem 273:17787-17792.

Eto T, Kitamura K, and Kato J. (1999) Biological and clinical roles of adrenomedullin in circulation control and cardiovascular diseases. Clin Exp Pharmacol Physiol 26:371-380.

Eto T, Kato J, and Kitamura K. (2003) Regulation of production and secretion of adrenomedullin in the cardiovascular system. Regul Pept 112:61-69.

Garayoa M, Martinez A, Lee S, Pio R, An WG, Neckers L, Trepel J, Montuenga LM, Ryan H, Johnson R, Gassmann M, and Cuttitta F. (2000) Hypoxa-inducible factor-1 (HIF-1) up-regulates adrenomedullin expression in human tumor cell lines during oxygen deprivation: a possible promotion mechanism of carcinogenesis. Mol Endocrinol 14:848-862.

Hague S, Zhang L, Oehler MK., Manek S, MacKenzie IZ, Bicknell R, and Rees MC. (2000) Expression of the hypoxically regulated angiogenic factor adrenomedullin correlates with uterine leiomyoma vascular density Clin. Cancer Res 6:2808-2814.

Hinson JP, Kapas S, and Smith DM. (2000) Adrenomedullin, a multifunctional regulatory peptide. Endocr Rev 21:138-167.

Hirata Y, Mitaka C, Sato K, Nagura T, Tsunoda Y, Amaha K, and Marumo F. (1996) Increased circulating adrenomedullin, a novel vasodilatory peptide, in sepsis. J Clin Endocrinol Metab 81:1449-1453.

Horio T, Nishikimi T, Yoshihara F, Nagaya N, Matsuo H, Takishita S, and Kangawa K. (1998) Production and secretion of adrenomedullin in cultured rat cardiac myocytes and nonmyocytes: stimulation by interleukin-1beta and tumor necrosis factor-alpha. Endocrinology 139:4576-4580.

Isumi Y, Minamino N, Katafuchi T, Yoshioka M, Tsuji T, Kangawa K, and Matsuo H. (1998a) Adrenomedullin production in fibroblasts: its possible function as a growth regulator of Swiss 3T3 cells. Endocrinology 139:2552-2563.

Isumi Y, Shoji H, Sugo S, Tochimoto T, Yoshioka M, Kangawa K, Matsuo H, and Minamino N. (1998b) Regulation of adrenomedullin production in rat endothelial cells. Endocrinology 139:838-846.

Jougasaki M, Wei CM, Heublein DM, Sandberg SM, and Burnett JC. (1995b) Immunohistochemical localization of adrenomedullin in canine heart and aorta. Peptides 16:773-775.

Kapas S, Martinez A, Cuttitta F, and Hinson JP. (1998) Local production and action of adrenomedullin in the rat adrenal zona glomerulosa. J Endocrinol 156:477-484.

Kapas S, Tenchini ML, and Farthing PM. (2001) Regulation of adrenomedullin secretion in cultured human skin and oral keratinocytes. J Invest Dermatol 117:353-359.

Kato H, Shichiri M, Marumo F, and Hirata Y. (1997) Adrenomedullin as an autocrine/paracrine apoptosis survival factor for rat endothelial cells. Endocrinology 138:2615-2620.

Kitamura K, Kangawa K, Kawamoto M, Ichiki Y, Nakamura S, Matsuo H, and Eto T. (1993) Adrenomedullin: a novel hypotensive peptide isolated from human pheochromocytoma. Biochem Biophys Res Commun 192:553-560.

Kitamura K, Kangawa K, and Eto T. (2002) Adrenomedullin and PAMP: discovery, structures, and cardiovascular functions. Microsc Res Tech 57: 3-13.

Kitamuro T, Takahashi K, Nakayama M, Murakami O, Hida W, Shirato K, and Shibahara S. (2000) Induction of adrenomedullin during hypoxia in cultured human glioblastoma cells J Neurochem 75:1826-1833.

Kobayashi H, Yamamoto R, Kitamura K, Niina H, Masumoto K, Minami SI, Yanagita T, Izumi F, Aunis D, Eto T, and Wada A. (1999) Cyclic AMP-dependent synthesis and release of adrenomedullin and PAMP in cultured bovine adrenal chromaffin cells. Eur J Biochem 263:702-708.

Kubo A, Minamino N, Isumi Y, Kangawa K, Dohi K, and Matsuo H. (1998a) Adrenomedullin production is correlated with differentiation in human leukemia cell lines and peripheral blood monocytes. FEBS Lett 426:233-237.

Kubo A, Minamino N, Isumi Y, Katafuchi T, Kangawa K, Dohi K, and Matsuo H. (1998b) Production of adrenomedullin in macrophage cell line and peritoneal macrophage. J Biol Chem 273:16730-16738.

Ladoux A, and Frelin C. (2000) Coordinated Up-regulation by hypoxia of adrenomedullin and one of its putative receptors (RDC-1) in cells of the rat blood-brain barrier J Biol Chem 275:39914-39919.

Lai KN, Leung JC, Yeung VT, Lewis LK, and Nicholls MG. (1998) Gene transcription and synthesis of adrenomedullin by cultured human renal cells. Biochem Biophys Res Commun 244:567-572.

Leonard MO, Cottell DC, Godson C, Brady HR, and Taylor CT. (2003) The role of HIF-1 alpha in transcriptional regulation of the proximal tubular epithelial cell response to hypoxia. J Biol Chem 278:40296-304.

Li Y, Totsune K, Takeda K, Furuyama K, Shibahara S, and Takahashi K. (2003) Differential expression of adrenomedullin and resistin in 3T3-L1 adipocytes treated with tumor necrosis factor-alpha. Eur J Endocrinol 149:231-238.

Ma Y, Freitag P, Zhou J, Brune B, Frede S, and Fandrey J. (2004) Thyroid hormone one induces erythropoietin gene expression through augmented accumulation of hypoxia-inducible factor-1. Am J Physiol in press.

Makino Y, Nakamura H, Ikeda E, Ohnuma K, Yamauchi K, Yabe Y, Poellinger L, Okada Y, Morimoto C, and Tanaka H. (2003) Hypoxia-inducible factor regulates survival of antigen receptor-driven T cells. J Immunol 171:6534-40.

Martinez A, Miller MJ, Unsworth EJ, Siegfried JM, and Cuttitta F. (1995) Expression of adrenomedullin in normal human lung and in pulmonary tumors. Endocrinology 136:4099-4105.

Marutsuka K, Hatakeyama K, Sato Y, Yamashita A, Sumiyoshi A, and Asada Y. (2003) Immunohistological localization and possible functions of adrenomedullin. Hypertens Res 26:S33-40.

Matsuzawa Y, Funahashi T, Kihara S, and Shimomura I. (2004) Adiponectin and metabolic syndrome. Arterioscler Thromb Vasc Biol 24:29-33.

Michibata H, Mukoyama M, Tanaka I, Suga S, Nakagawa M, Ishibashi R, Goto M, Akaji K, Fujiwara Y, Kiso Y. and Nakao K. (1998) Autocrine/paracrine role of adrenomedullin in cultured endothelial and mesangial cells. Kidney Int 53:979-985.

Minamino N, Kikumoto K, and Isumi Y. (2002) Regulation of adrenomedullin expression and release. Microsc Res Tech 57: 28-39.

Moriyama T, Otani T, and Maruo T. (2000) Expression of adrenomedullin by human granulosa lutein cells and its effect on progesterone production. Eur J Endocrinol 142:671-676.

Nagata D, Hirata Y, Suzuki E, Kakoki M, Hayakawa H, Goto A, Ishimitsu T, Minamino N, Ono Y, Kangawa K, Matsuo H, and Omata M. (1999) Hypoxia-induced adrenomedullin production in the kidney. Kidney Int 55:1259-1267.

Nakayama M, Takahashi K, Murakami O, Shirato K, and Shibahara S. (1999a) Induction of adrenomedullin by hypoxia in cultured human coronary artery endothelial cells. Peptides 20:769-772.

Nakayama M, Takahashi K, Murakami O, Yanai M, Sasaki H, Shirato K, and Shibahara S. (1999b) Production and secretion of adrenomedullin in cultured human alveolar macrophages. Peptides 20:1123-1125.

Nishikimi T, Yoshihara F, Horinaka S, Kobayashi N, Mori Y, Tadokoro K, Akimoto K, Minamino N, Kangawa K, and Matsuoka H. (2003) Chronic administration of adrenomedullin attenuates transition from left ventricular hypertrophy to heart failure in rats. Hypertension 42:1034-1041.

Nishimura J, Seguchi H, Sakihara C, Kureishi Y, Yoshimura H, Kobayashi S, and Kanaide H. (1997) The relaxant effect of adrenomedullin on particular smooth muscles despite a general expression of its mRNA in smooth muscle, endothelial and epithelial cells. Br J Pharmacol 120:193-200.

Nishio K, Akai Y, Murao Y, Doi N, Ueda S, Tabuse H, Miyamoto S, Dohi K, Minamino N, Shoji H, Kitamura K, Kangawa K, and Matsuo H. (1997) Increased plasma concentrations of adrenomedullin correlate with relaxation of vascular tone in patients with septic shock. Crit Care Med 25:953-957.

Niu P, Shindo T, Iwata H, Iimuro S, Takeda N, Zhang Y, Ebihara A, Suematsu Y, Kangawa K, Hirata Y, and Nagai R. (2004) Protective effects of endogenous adrenomedullin on cardiac hypertrophy, fibrosis, and renal damage. Circulation 109:1789-1794.

Oehler MK, Norbury C, Hague S, Rees MC, and Bicknell R. (2001) Adrenomedullin inhibits hypoxic cell death by upregulation of Bcl-2 in endometrial cancer cells: a possible promotion mechanism for tumour growth. Oncogene 20:2937-2945.

Pewitt EB, Haleem R, and Wang Z. (1999) Adrenomedullin gene is abundantly expressed and directly regulated by androgen in the rat ventral prostate. Endocrinology 140:2382-2386.

Sandner P, Hofbauer KH, Tinel H, Kurtz A, Thiesson HC, Ottosen PD, Walter S, Skott O, and Jensen BL. (2004) Expression of adrenomedullin in hypoxic and ischemic rat kidneys and human kidneys with arterial stenosis. Am J Physiol 286:R942-951.

Sato K, Imai T, Iwashina M, Marumo F, and Hirata Y. (1998) Secretion of adrenomedullin by renal tubular cell lines. Nephron 78:9-14.

Shimosawa T, Ogihara T, Matsui H, Asano T, Ando K, and Fujita T. (2003) Deficiency of adrenomedullin induces insulin resistance by increasing oxidative stress. Hypertension 41:1080-1085.

Shindo T, Kurihara H, Maemura K, Kurihara Y, Kuwaki T, Izumida T, Minamino N, Ju KH, Morita H, Oh-hashi Y, Kumada M, Kangawa K, Nagai R, and Yazaki Y. (2000b) Hypotension and resistance to lipopolysaccharide-induced shock in transgenic mice overexpressing adrenomedullin in their vasculature. Circulation 101:2309-2316.

Shinoki N, Kawasaki T, Minamino N, Okahara K, Ogawa A, Ariyoshi H, Sakon M, Kambayashi J, Kangawa K, and Monden M. (1998) Shear stress down-regulates gene transcription and production of adrenomedullin in human aortic endothelial cells. J Cell Biochem 71:109-115.

Shoji H, Minamino N, Kangawa K, and Matsuo H. (1995) Endotoxin markedly elevates plasma concentration and gene transcription of adrenomedullin in the rat. Biochem Biophys Res Commun 215:531-537.

Sugo S, Minamino N, Kangawa K, Miyamoto K, Kitamura K, Sakata J, Eto T, and Matsuo H. (1994a) Endothelial cells actively synthesize and secrete adrenomedullin. Biochem Biophys Res Commun 201:1160-1166.

Sugo S, Minamino N, Shoji H, Kangawa K, Kitamura K, Eto T, and Matsuo H. (1994b) Production and secretion of adrenomedullin from vascular smooth muscle cells: augmented production by tumor necrosis factor-alpha. Biochem Biophys Res Commun 203:719-726.

Sugo S, Minamino N, Shoji H, Kangawa K, Kitamura K, Eto T, and Matsuo H. (1995a) Interleukin-1, tumor necrosis factor and lipopolysaccharide additively stimulate production of adrenomedullin in vascular smooth muscle cells. Biochem Biophys Res Commun 207:25-32.

Takahashi K, Satoh F, Hara E, Sone M, Murakami O, Kayama T, Yoshimoto T, and Shibahara S. (1997) Production and secretion of adrenomedullin from glial cell tumors and its effects on cAMP production. Peptides 18:1117-1124.

Takahashi K, Nakayama M, Totsune K, Murakami O, Sone M, Kitamuro T, Yoshinoya A, and Shibahara S. (2000a) Increased secretion of adrenomedullin from cultured human astrocytes by cytokines. J

Neurochem 74:99-103.
Takahashi K, Yoshinoya A, Murakami O, Totsune K, and Shibahara S. (2000b) Production and secretion of two vasoactive peptides, adrenomedullin and endothelin-1, by cultured human adrenocortical carcinoma cells. Peptides 21:251-256.
Tomoda Y, Kikumoto K, Isumi Y, Katafuchi T, Tanaka A, Kangawa K, Dohi K, and Minamino N. (2001a) Cardiac fibroblasts are major production and target cells of adrenomedullin in the heart in vitro. Cardiovasc Res 49:721-730.
Tomoda Y, Isumi Y, Katafuchi T, and Minamino N. (2001b) Regulation of adrenomedullin secretion from cultured cells. Peptides 22: 1783-1794.
Tsuruda T, Kato J, Kitamura K, Kuwasako K, Imamura T, Koiwaya Y, Tsuji T, Kangawa K, and Eto T. (1998) Adrenomedullin: a possible autocrine or paracrine inhibitor of hypertrophy of cardiomyocytes. Hypertension 31:505-510.
Tsuruda T, Kato J, Kitamura K, Kawamoto M, Kuwasako K, Imamura T, Koiwaya Y, Tsuji T, Kangawa K, and Eto T. (1999) An autocrine or a paracrine role of adrenomedullin in modulating cardiac fibroblast growth. Cardiovasc Res 43:958-967.
Udono T, Takahashi K, Nakayama M, Yoshinoya A, Totsune K, Murakami O, Durlu YK, Tamai M, and Shibahara S. (2001) Induction of adrenomedullin by hypoxia in cultured retinal pigment epithelial cells. Invest Ophthalmol Vis Sci 42:1080-6.
Ueda S, Nishio K, Minamino N, Kubo A, Akai Y, Kangawa K, Matsuo H, Fujimura Y, Yoshioka A, Masui K, Doi N, Murao Y, and Miyamoto S. (1999) Increased plasma levels of adrenomedullin in patients with systemic inflammatory response syndrome. Am J Respir Crit Care Med 160:132-136.
Yin H, Chao L, and Chao J. (2004) Adrenomedullin protects against myocardial apoptosis after ischemia/reperfusion through activation of Akt-GSK signaling. Hypertension 43:109-116.
Yoshibayashi M, Kamiya T, Nishikimi T, Saito Y, Matsuo H, and Kangawa K. (1999) Elevated plasma levels of adrenomedullin in congenital cyanotic heart disease. Clin Sci (Lond) 96:543-547.

5

BIOLOGICAL ACTION OF ADRENOMEDULLIN

Takeshi Horio and Fumiki Yoshihara

Department of Medicine, National Cardiovascular Center, Osaka, Japan

INTRODUCTION

Adrenomedullin (AM) was originally described as a powerful vasodilatory peptide, and its biological actions have been mainly focused on the cardiovascular system. However, subsequent studies have revealed that AM also has a remarkable range of actions in the central nervous, endocrine, digestive, reproductive, and immune systems and other various organs and tissues (Hinson et al., 2000; Beltowski and Jamroz, 2004).

1. VASCULATURE

Systemic administration of AM elicits a potent hypotensive effect due to its vasodilatory action. The hemodynamic effects of human AM were initially investigated in anesthetized rats (Kitamura et al., 1993). Intravenous bolus injection of AM caused a rapid, remarkable, and long-lasting reduction in blood pressure in a dose-dependent manner. The maximum decrease in mean blood pressure after injection of a high dose (3 nmol/kg) of AM was approximately 50 mmHg, and the significant hypotensive effect lasted for 30-60 minutes. The reduction in blood pressure was closely associated with the decrease in total peripheral resistance, and this was concomitant with increases in cardiac output and stroke volume, probably secondary to reduced afterload (Ishimaya et al., 1993). In their study using anesthetized rats, heart rate was not significantly altered by AM injection. However, many other studies showed that reflex tachycardia in response to blood pressure fall was observed. The hypotensive effect of AM was also seen in both conscious and hypertensive rats. In addition, a significant decrease in systemic blood pressure induced by acute or chronic administration of AM has been observed in rabbit, sheep, and human. Furthermore, vasodilatory actions of AM have been studied in not only the systemic vasculature but also regional vascular beds including renal (Hirata et al., 1995), pulmonary (Lippton et al., 1994), cerebral (Lang et al., 1997), and coronary circulation (Yoshimoto et al., 1998).

Many studies have addressed the mechanism of vasodilatory effect of AM and the results differ depending on animal species and vascular preparation. Most observations indicate that AM may induce endothelium-independent relaxation by acting on calcitonin gene-related peptide (CGRP) receptors and elevating cAMP level in vascular smooth muscle cells (Eguchi et al., 1994). For example, in perfused rat mesenteric vascular beds, administration of AM induced endothelium-independent vasodilation. This vasodilator response was not affected by atropine or propranolol, but was clearly inhibited by CGRP(8-37), an antagonist for CGRP1 receptor, suggesting that AM induced nonadrenergic and noncholinergic vasodilation in which CGRP receptors might be involved (Nuki et al., 1993). On the other hand, AM binds to specific receptors in endothelial cells and elicits endothelium-dependent vasorelaxation mediated by nitric oxide. Shimekake et al. (1995) minutely investigated the biological action of AM on cultured bovine aortic endothelial cells. According to their study, the specific binding of AM to endothelial cells was observed, and AM induced intracellular cAMP accumulation in a dose-dependent manner. AM also induced an increase in intracellular free Ca in endothelial cells in a dose-dependent manner. This intracellular free Ca increase resulted from phospholipase C activation and inositol 1,4,5-trisphosphate formation, and seemed to cause nitric oxide synthase activation by monitoring intracellular cGMP accumulation. As another mechanism of endothelial nitric oxide synthase activation by AM, Nishimatsu et al. (2001) showed that phosphatidylinositol 3-kinase/Akt pathway was involved. In addition, endothelium-derived hyperpolarizing factor, vasodilatory prostanoids, and suppressed production of endothelin-1 may be implicated in AM-induced endothelium-dependent vasorelaxation. Taken together, it is proper that the vasodilatory effect of AM is mediated by at least two mechanisms, a direct action on vascular smooth muscle cells and an indirect effect through primary actions on endothelial cells.

AM clearly inhibits platelet-derived growth factor- or angiotensin II-induced migration of vascular smooth muscle cells (Horio et al., 1995). In addition to the antimigratory effect, AM also inhibits vascular smooth muscle cell proliferation stimulated by serum or platelet-derived growth factor (Kano et al., 1996). In quiescent cells, however, AM has been shown to elicit a growth-promoting effect (Iwasaki et al., 1998). Therefore, AM may bidirectionally regulate the proliferation of vascular smooth muscle cells. As for other direct effects on those cells, AM inhibits endothelin-1 production and stimulates inducible nitric oxide synthase in cultured rat aortic smooth muscle cells.

AM inhibits serum deprivation-induced endothelial cell apoptosis via a cAMP-independent mechanism (Kato et al., 1997). In addition, AM has been recently shown to promote endothelial regeneration and angiogenesis through Akt activation (Miyashita et al., 2003; Kim et al., 2003). Taken together with several recent findings concerning protective roles of AM against acute ischemia and vascular injury (Abe et al., 2003; Kawai et al., 2004), there may be a possibility that AM is useful as a novel therapeutic strategy for some kinds of vascular disease.

2. HEART

Systemic administration of AM markedly increases cardiac output in both normal men and patients with congestive heart failure (Lainchbury et al., 2000; Nagaya et al., 2000), and this effect appears to be mainly due to reduced peripheral resistance. There are discrepant findings as to the direct effect of AM on myocardial contractility. Ikenouchi et al. (1997) have demonstrated that AM has a negative inotropic action in isolated adult rabbit ventricular myocytes through cAMP-independent and nitric oxide/cGMP-dependent pathway. In contrast, AM has been shown to have positive inotropic effects on the heart of rats via cAMP-dependent or independent mechanism (Ihara et al., 2000; Szokodi et al., 1998), or to have no significant effects on myocardial contractility (Stangl et al., 2000).

It is currently known that AM inhibits angiotensin II- and phenylephrine-induced hypertrophy of cultured ventricular myocytes (Tsuruda et al., 1998). In addition, AM strongly inhibits DNA and extracellular matrix production in cultured cardiac fibroblasts, suggesting that AM may play a role as a regulator of cardiac remodeling (Horio et al., 1999). AM has also been revealed to inhibit cardiomyocyte apoptosis induced by doxorubicin

(Tokudome et al., 2002) and ischemia/reperfusion injury (Yin et al., 2004).

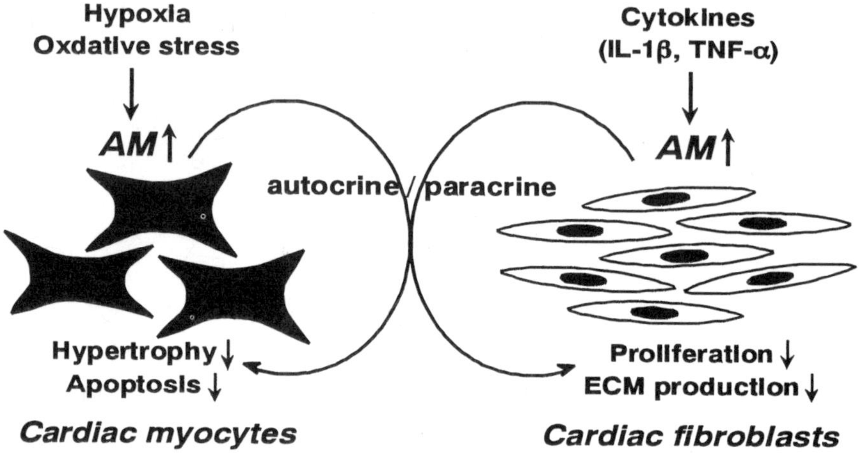

Figure 1. Autocrine and paracrine effects of AM secreted from cardiac myocytes and fibroblasts. ECM, extracellular matrix.

AM is synthesized and secreted from cardiac myocytes and fibroblasts, and its production is up-regulated by stimulations such as hypoxia, oxidative stress, and several cytokines in those cells, respectively (Yoshihara et al., 2002; Horio et al., 1998). On the basis of these observations and the protective effects of endogenous AM against angiotensin II-induced cardiac hypertrophy and fibrosis (Niu et al., 2004) and oxidative stress-mediated cardiac damage (Shimosawa T et al., 2002), AM may play an important role as an autocrine or paracrine modulator in some cardiac disorders (Figure 1).

3. KIDNEY

AM and its gene expression have been reported to be observed in the glomerulus, distal tubules, and medullary collecting duct cells of the kidney (Asada et al., 1999). McLatchie et al. (1998) demonstrated that the calcitonin receptor-like receptor (CRLR), a receptor with 7 transmembrane domains, can function as either a CGRP receptor or an AM receptor, depending on which members of a new family of single-transmembrane-domain proteins, which are called receptor-activity-modifying proteins

(RAMPs), are expressed. RAMP1 presents the receptor at the cell surface as a CGRP receptor, whereas RAMP2- or RAMP3-transported receptors are AM. CRLR, RAMP2, and RAMP3 mRNAs were expressed in the rat renal cortex and medulla (Yoshihara et al., 2001). Immunohistochemical analysis of the human kidney revealed CRLR-like immunoreactivity in the juxtaglomerular arteries, the glomerular capillaries and chief cells of the collecting duct (Hagner et al., 2002). These results suggest that AM and its receptor system in the kidney may be involved in the regulation of renal hemodynamics, glomerular filtration and tubular Na^+ homeostasis in vivo.

There is also evidence for a role for AM in mesangial cell biology. Mesangial cells grown in primary culture synthesize AM which is stimulated by TNF alpha (Lai et al., 1998) and IL-1 beta (Chini et al., 1997) and under hypoxic conditions (Nagata et al., 1999). AM increases cAMP levels in mesangial cells (Kohno et al., 1995) leading to inhibited proliferation (Michibata et al., 1998), reactive oxygen generation and macrophage infiltration (Chini et al., 1997). In addition, AM has been reported to stimulate hyalurnoic acid, an important extracellular matrix component, release from mesangial cells through p38 kinase and PI3-kinase pathways (Parameswaran et al., 1999). These data suggest that there may be a role for AM not only in the pathophysiology of mesangial cell proliferation and matrix biology, but also in protecting the renal glomeruli from inflammatory reactions or immune injuries.

Although AM mRNA expression has been reported to exist in glomerulus, cortical collecting duct, outer medullary collecting duct, and inner medullary collecting duct (Owada et al., 1997), it is still unclear whether AM directly regulates tubular transport. AM increases cAMP levels in renal tubular basolateral membranes (Osajima et al., 1995) and the cortical thick ascending limb, and in the distal convoluted tubule (Edwards et al., 1996). These data suggest that AM may have an autocrine/paracrine role in renal tubular function. AM stimulates osmotic water permeability in the inner medullary collecting duct (Owada et al., 1997) and Na^+ uptake in apical membranes of the distal tubules (Leclerc and Brunette, 2000). These effects would favor activation of tubular reabsorption, although AM is known to be a natriuretic hormone probably through its vasodilating action.

Intravenous infusion of AM in healthy volunteers (Lainchbury et al., 2000) resulted in an increase in plasma renin activity associated with a decrease in arterial blood pressure. Jensen et al. (1997) reported that AM is expressed in juxtaglomerular structures and that it has a direct stimulatory effect on renin secretion and renin mRNA abundance by receptors on juxtaglomerular cells, possibly through increases in cAMP. AM may act as an autocrine/paracrine stimulatory factor in the control of renin secretion and renin gene expression.

AM administration to experimental animals has been reported to increase urine output and urinary sodium excretion in a dose-dependent manner (Ebara et al., 1994) in association with renal vasodilation, increased in renal blood flow, and glomerular filtration rate (GFR). However, as low doses of AM increase natriuresis without affecting GFR, AM may inhibit tubular sodium reabsorption (Nagaya et al., 1999). AM-induced renal vasodilator, diuretic, and natriuretic responses may be partially mediated by the release of endogenous nitric oxide (Majid et al., 1996) and renal prostaglandins (Jougasaki et al., 1997). Interestingly, neutral endopeptidase (NEP) inhibition potentiates an increase in sodium excretion in the absence of an increase in GFR or further increases in renal blood flow in response to exogenous AM (Lisy et al., 1998), indicating not only that AM may be a substrate for NEP, but also that a decrease in tubular sodium reabsorption may be the mechanism for natriuresis.

4. ENDOCRINE

(1) Pituitary

AM immunoreactivity has been detected in the hypothalamo-pituitary-adrenal axis of humans, rats, and pigs (Nussdorfer et al., 1997), suggesting that AM may have a role in modulating the secretion of pituitary and adrenal hormones. AM inhibits basal and corticotropin releasing hormone (CRH)-stimulated ACTH secretion from dispersed, rat anterior pituitary cells in a significant, dose-related fashion (Samson et al., 1995). Intravenous infusion of human AM also decreases plasma ACTH levels in conscious, chronically instrumented sheep (Parkes and May, 1995). These studies suggest that AM has a role in inhibiting ACTH release. In contrast, intracerebroventricular infusion of AM significantly increases plasma ACTH level in conscious rats, in association with increased Fos expression in neurons within autonomic centers including the paraventricular nucleus (PVN) of the hypothalamus (Shan and Krukoff, 2001). In the PVN, large proportions of CRF- and nitric oxide-producing neurons were activated (Fos positive). These data suggest that intracerebroventricular AM stimulates the hypothalamo-pituitary-adrenal axis by activating CRH-producing neurons. These contrasting findings suggest that the effects of AM on the hypothalamo-pituitary-adrenal axis may vary according to the site of action. Regarding the relationship between AM and other anterior pituitary hormones, previous reports demonstrated that (1) AM was a growth hormone secretagogue in human and rat pituitary somatotrophs (Nakamura et al., 1998); (2) intravenous infusion of AM in healthy volunteers increases plasma PRL level (Meeran et al., 1997); (3) plasma AM levels correlated with serum free thyroid hormone levels in thyrotoxicosis (Taniyama et al., 1997); and (4) the changes in plasma AM were related to changes in LH during the menstrual cycle (Marinoni et al., 2000), suggesting that AM is involved in the regulation of production and release of these hormones. Concerning the posterior pituitary hormones, AM stimulates oxytocin (Serino et al., 1999) and inhibits hyperosmolality-stimulated vasopressin secretion (Yokoi et al., 1996). Intracerebroventricular AM infusion activates the neurosecretory cells in the PVN and supraoptic nuclei via specific AM receptors, and its infusion stimulates the secretion of oxytocin by activating hypothalamic oxytocin-producing cells (Serino et al., 1999).

(2) Adrenal gland

The regulatory effect of AM on aldosterone production and secretion in zona glomerulosa (ZG) cells is also remains controversial. AM inhibits aldosterone production induced by angiotensin II (Andreis et al., 1997a), potassium (Mazzocchi et al., 1999), and Ca^{2+} ionophores (Yamaguchi et al., 1995) in dispersed ZG cells. In vivo, AM has been reported to prevent an increase in plasma aldosterone level induced by infusion of angiotensin II (Petrie et al., 2000), a sodium-deficient diet or bilateral nephrectomy (Yamaguchi et al., 1996). These data suggest that AM may have an inhibitory role in secreting aldosterone from ZG cells. However, other reports demonstrated that AM increases basal aldosterone secretion via mediated by specific AM receptors coupled to adenylate cyclase, and that

AM had no effect on the response of ZG cells to stimulation by either ACTH or angiotensin II (Kapas et al., 1998). One possible reason for these contradictory data might be the stimulatory effect of aldosterone by catecholamines which were released from adrenal medullary cells induced by AM. Andreis et al. (1997b) investigated whether human AM exerts a modulatory action on steroid secretion of human dispersed adrenocortical cells (obtained from the gland tail deprived of chromaffin cells) and adrenal slices (including both capsule and medulla). AM exerts a direct inhibitory effect on angiotensin II-stimulated aldosterone secretion, which is overcome and reversed by an indirect stimulatory action, conceivably involving the release of catecholamines by adrenal chromaffin cells. In contrast to ZG cells, AM and its receptor system exists in the zona fasciculata and zona reticularis (ZF/R). These cultures were actually a mixture of ZG, ZF/R and medullary chromaffin cells. AM stimulates adrenomedullary cells to release catecholamines, which are able to enhance aldosterone secretion from ZG cells (Ziolkowska et al., 2003).

Apart from regulating hormone secretion, AM stimulates cell proliferation in the rat ZG. This mitogenic effect of AM is mediated by activation of the tyrosine kinase - mitogen-activated protein kinase cascade (Andreis et al., 2000). Prolonged (48-72 h) suppression of AM gene transcription by a specific antisense oligonucleotide or the long-lasting (24-96 h) blockade of AM receptors by a selective antagonist AM(22-52) significantly lowered the proliferation index and increased the apoptotic index of cultured ZG cells (Malendowicz et al., 2003), suggesting that the endogenous AM system may act as a physiological ZG growth regulator.

(3) Pancreas

With respect to the effect of AM on the pancreas, previous reports demonstrated that AM stimulates insulin release from isolated rat islets in the presence of glucose (Mulder et al., 1996). However, others reported that AM inhibits insulin secretion in a dose-dependent manner from isolated rat islets, that the neutralizing AM antibody increases insulin release and that intravenous injection of AM reduces the levels of insulin in the bloodstream with a concomitant increase in circulating glucose after an oral glucose tolerance test (Martinez et al., 1996). Although the reason for these opposing results is still unknown, a recent report demonstrated that AM may be not only a factor in maintaining insulin homeostasis and normoglycemia, but also a possible causal agent in diabetes. Zudaire et al. (2003a) reported that AM inhibits insulin secretion both in vitro (isolated rat islets) and in vivo (oral glucose tolerance test in rats) in a dose-dependent manner and that AM is elevated in plasma from patients with pancreatic dysfunctions such as type 1 or type 2 diabetes and insulinoma. Using a diabetic model in rats, they have shown that AM increases circulating glucose levels whereas a blocking monoclonal antibody against AM has the opposite effect and improves postprandial recovery.

(4) Reproductive effects

AM is produced by granulosa cells of the ovarian follicle (Abe et al., 1998). AM causes a dose-dependent increase in the intracellular levels of cAMP and enhances the effects of FSH, acting additionally to produce cAMP in the granulosa cells (Marinoni et al., 2002). Since FSH in known to induce granulosa cell differentiation through cAMP-mechanism, AM may play a supportive role in the process of granulosa cell differentiation. In patients undergoing ovarian stimulation, follicular fluid AM levels correlated with serum 17beta-estradiol concentration, suggesting a possible regulatory effect of the sexual hormones on AM production by the ovary during the ovulatory process (Marinoni et al., 2002). AM levels in follicular fluid collected just before ovulation were significantly higher than those in the plasma. Furthermore, addition of AM to cultured granulosa lutein cells augmented progesterone secretion in a dose-dependent manner, suggesting AM may be a local factor to enhance progesterone production by granulosa lutein cells (Moriyama et al., 2000). Plasma AM levels increase during the follicular phase and decrease during the luteal phase of the menstrual cycle, and the changes in plasma AM are related to changes in LH and 17beta-estradiol (Marinoni et al., 2000). These data suggest that AM may be involved in the regulation of fluid and electrolyte homeostasis during the menstrual cycle.

5. CENTRAL NERVOUS SYSTEM

AM immunoreactivity is detected in many neurons throughout the brain and spinal cord. In particular, abundant levels of AM are expressed in the thalamus, hypothalamus, and hypophysis. One of the hypothalamic functions is to control feeding and drinking behavior, and AM has been shown to be importantly involved in the regulation of food and water intake. Taylor et al. (1996) reported that intracerebroventricular administration of AM caused a dose-dependent decrease in 2-hour food intake in fasted rats. Murphy and Samson (1995) showed that cerebroventricular injection of AM suppressed pharmacologically induced (central administration of angiotensin II) water drinking and also had an inhibitory effect on physiologically induced (overnight water deprivation) water drinking in rats. No significant change in blood pressure, heart rate, or motor activity supported that the observed inhibitory effects of AM were direct central actions, independent of a certain effect on cardiovascular function or locomotion. The same study group also demonstrated that centrally administered AM significantly attenuated saline drinking in response to isotonic hypovolemia. These effects on water drinking and salt appetite suggest that AM may act within the central nervous system to determine fluid and electrolyte balance, in addition to its peripheral actions on cardiovascular and renal function.

Some studies have revealed the central actions of AM on gastric function. Intracisternal injection of AM or CGRP dose-dependently inhibits gastric emptying in conscious rats, and the inhibitory effects of AM and CGRP are completely blocked by CGRP(8-37), but not by corticotropin-releasing factor receptor antagonist (Martinez et al., 1997). In addition, the central AM action is abolished by bilateral adrenalectomy or the beta-adrenergic blocker, propranolol, but not altered by indomethacin or subdiaphragmatic vagotomy. These observations indicate that centrally administered AM inhibits gastric emptying through adrenal-dependent, beta-adrenergic pathways independently from activation of central corticotropin-releasing factor receptors. Intracerebroventricular administration of AM is also shown to prevent reserpine-induced gastric ulcers in rats, being mediated via CGRP receptors (Clementi et al., 1998).

In conscious rats, centrally injected AM increases urine output and urinary sodium and potassium excretion, indicating that some central AM actions correspond with its peripheral effects. The central action of AM on systemic

blood pressure, however, has shown to present a striking contrast to the hypotensive effect of AM in the periphery. Therefore, central administration of AM elevates blood pressure and heart rate in both anesthetized (Takahashi et al., 1994) and conscious, unrestrained rats (Saita et al., 1998). Pretreatment with antagonists CGRP(8-37) and AM(22-52) significantly suppressed the central hypertensive actions of AM. In these studies using anesthetized and conscious rats, changes in sympathetic nerve activities in relation to the blood pressure elevation were observed. These findings suggest that AM, as a neuropeptide, contributes to the receptor-mediated central regulation of the cardiovascular system. Such central hypertensive and sympathostimulatory actions of AM may be cardioprotective; e.g., it functions against cardiovascular collapse during septic shock.
The role of AM in brain ischemia has been studied. Wang et al. (1995) demonstrated using a focal stroke rat model by middle cerebral artery occlusion that both AM mRNA and its immunoreactivity were remarkably up-regulated in ischemic cortical neurons. They also showed that intracerebroventricular AM administration prior to and after artery occlusion, increased the degree of focal ischemic injury, suggesting the possibility that vasodilating effects of AM on cerebral vessels exacerbate ischemic brain damage. In contrast, Dogan et al. (1997) showed using the same ischemic model of spontaneously hypertensive rats that intravenous AM infusion decreased the degree of ischemic brain injury, and they concluded AM may play a role in preventing ischemic brain damage by increasing collateral circulation.

6. OTHERS

(1) Lung

In addition to pulmonary vasodilatory effects, AM inhibits histamine- or acetylcholine-induced bronchoconstriction in anesthetized guinea pigs (Kanazawa et al., 1994). Since plasma levels of AM are reported to rise during an acute asthma attack, AM may play an important role in airway function. Furthermore, AM may have an antiinflammatory role in the lung, because a previous study showed that AM significantly inhibited the secretion of cytokine-induced neutrophil chemoattractant, a member of the interleukin-8 family, from lipopolysaccharide-stimulated rat alveolar macrophages (Kamoi et al., 1995).

(2) Digestive apparatus

AM mRNA and AM immunoreactivity are detected in gastrointestinal mucosa, and gastrointestinal AM gene expression is up-regulated by fasting. Intravenous administration of AM inhibits both basal and gastrin-stimulated gastric acid secretion in conscious rats (Rossowski et al., 1997). In addition, AM prevents damage of gastric mucosa in either reserpine-treated or pylorus-ligated rats (Salomone et al., 2003). Taken together with the central actions of AM on gastric function (described above), AM is thought to have an anti-ulcer effect through the inhibition of gastric acid secretion.
AM and its specific binding sites are also localized in the pancreas and liver. AM inhibits stimulated amylase secretion by reducing the calcium sensitivity of the exocytotic machinery of the pancreatic acini (Tsuchida et al., 1999). In addition, AM contributes to the relaxation of hepatic stellate cells and the regulation of sinusoidal microcirculation (Kawada and Inoue, 1994).

(3) Bone

Expression of AM, and its receptor are seen in osteoblasts during the later stages of rodent embryogenesis and in maturing chrondocytes of fetal mice. AM stimulates the proliferation of fetal and adult rat osteoblasts. Also, AM increases protein synthesis in vitro and mineralized and bone area in vivo (Cornish et al., 1997). Another study demonstrated that human osteoblasts secrete immunoreactive AM and that AM stimulates intracellular cAMP production in these cells, suggesting the role of endogenous AM as an autocrine or paracrine regulator of bone formation (Hamada et al., 2002).

(4) Reproductive organs

AM stimulates uterine growth and vascularization (Zhao et al., 1998), and inhibits spontaneous and bradykinin-induced uterine contractility (Yanagita et al., 2000). A marked increase in plasma AM concentration is observed during pregnancy, and this increase may be related to the production of AM by the uterus and placenta. In addition, AM is detected in amniotic fluid at higher levels than in plasma. Although the physiological significance of AM in pregnancy has not been sufficiently clarified, AM may play various roles during normal pregnancy. For example, AM may contribute to maternal hemodynamic changes and regulation of local uteroplacental circulation. AM may also be importantly involved in embryogenesis and differentiation, placental development, and placental vasculogenesis (Montuenga et al., 1997; Beltowski and Jamroz, 2004).

(5) Immunity and inflammation

The epithelium provides a first line of defense against potentially pathogenic microorganisms. AM is produced by epithelial cells at mucosal surfaces, such as skin, oral cavity, and respiratory and gastrointestinal tract, and AM has antimicrobial properties against both Gram-positive and Gram-negative bacteria in these spots (Allaker et al., 1999). AM has also been shown to stimulate proliferation and inhibit apoptosis of cultured immature rat thymocytes, suggesting AM may play a role in the development of immunity (Belloni et al., 2003).
AM gene is expressed in peripheral blood monocytes and is rapidly up-regulated during their transformation to macrophages. Some studies showed that AM suppresses the secretion of proinflammatory cytokines such as tumor necrosis factor-α in Swiss 3T3 cells, macrophage cell line, and rat Kupffer cells (Isumi et al., 1999; Wu et al., 2003). The antiinflammatory effect of AM was also demonstrated in different in vivo models of inflammation (Clementi et al., 1999).

(6) Neoplasm

AM was originally purified from human pheochromocytoma, an adrenal tumor (Kitamura et al., 1993). Subsequent studies have shown that AM and its receptors are expressed in many types of tumor cells. In addition, AM exerts mitogenic effects on some types of tumor cells (Miller et al., 1996). These findings suggest the possibility that AM acts as an autocrine/paracrine growth factor in tumors (Zudaire et al., 2003b).

REFERENCES

Abe K, Minegishi T, Tano M, Hirakawa T, Tsuchiya M, Kangawa K, Kojima M, and Ibuki Y. (1998) Expression and effect of adrenomedullin on rat granulosa cell. Endocrinology 139:5263-5266.

Abe M, Sata M, Nishimatsu H, Nagata D, Suzuki E, Terauchi Y, Kadowaki T, Minamino N, Kangawa K, Matsuo H, Hirata Y, and Nagai R. (2003) Adrenomedullin augments collateral development in response to acute ischemia. Biochem Biophys Res Commun 306:10-15.

Allaker RP, Zihni C, and Kapas S. (1999) An investigation into the antimicrobial effects of adrenomedullin on members of the skin, oral, respiratory tract and gut microflora. FEMS Immunol Med Microbiol 23:289-293.

Andreis PG, Markowska A, Champion HC, Mazzocchi G, Malendowicz LK, and Nussdorfer GG. (2000) Adrenomedullin enhances cell proliferation and deoxyribonucleic acid synthesis in rat adrenal zona glomerulosa: receptor subtype involved and signaling mechanism. Endocrinology 141:2098-2104.

Andreis PG, Mazzocchi G, Rebuffat P, and Nussdorfer GG. (1997a) Effects of adrenomedullin and proadrenomedullin N-terminal 20 peptide on rat zona glomerulosa cells. Life Sci 60:1693-1697.

Andreis PG, Neri G, Prayer GT, Rossi GP, Gottardo G, Malendowicz LK, and Nussdorfer GG. (1997b) Effects of adrenomedullin on the human adrenal glands: an in vitro study. J Clin Endocrinol Metab 82:1167-1170.

Asada Y, Hara S, Marutsuka K, Kitamura K, Tsuji T, Sakata J, Sato Y, Kisanuki A, Eto T, and Sumiyoshi A. (1999) Novel distribution of adrenomedullin-immunoreactive cells in human tissues. Histochem Cell Biol 112:185-191.

Belloni AS, Trejter M, Malendowicz LK, and Nussdorfer GG. (2003) Adrenomedullin stimulates proliferation and inhibits apoptosis of immature rat thymocytes cultured in vitro. Peptides 24:295-300.

Beltowski J and Jamroz A. (2004) Adrenomedullin - what we know 10 years since its discovery? Pol J Pharmacol 56:5-27.

Chini EN, Chini CC, Bolliger C, Jougasaki M, Grande JP, Burnett JC Jr, and Dousa TP. (1997) Cytoprotective effects of adrenomedullin in glomerular cell injury: central role of cAMP signaling pathway. Kidney Int 52:917-925.

Clementi G, Caruso A, Cutuli VMC, deBernardis E, Prato A, Mangano NG, and Amico-Roxas M. (1998) Effects of centrally or peripherally injected adrenomedullin on reserpine-induced gastric lesions. Eur J Pharmacol 360:51-54.

Clementi G, Caruso A, Cutuli VM, Prato A, Mangano NG, and Amico-Roxas M. (1999) Antiinflammatory activity of adrenomedullin in the acetic acid peritonitis in rats. Life Sci 65:PL203-PL208.

Cornish J, Callon KE, Coy DH, Jiang NY, Xiao L, Cooper GJ, and Reid IR. (1997) Adrenomedullin is a potent stimulator of osteoblastic activity in vitro and in vivo. Am J Physiol 273:E1113-E1120.

Dogan A, Suzuki Y, Koketsu N, Osuka K, Saito K, Takayasu M, Shibuya M, and Yoshida J. (1997) Intravenous infusion of adrenomedullin and increase in regional cerebral blood flow and prevention of ischemic brain injury after middle cerebral artery occlusion in rats. J Cereb Blood Flow Metab 17:19-25.

Ebara T, Miura K, Okumura M, Matsuura T, Kim S, Yukimura T, and Iwao H. (1994) Effect of adrenomedullin on renal hemodynamics and functions in dogs. Eur J Pharmacol 263:69-73.

Edwards RM, Trizna W, Stack E, and Aiyar N. (1996) Effect of adrenomedullin on cAMP levels along the rat nephron: comparison with CGRP. Am J Physiol 271:F895-F899.

Eguchi S, Hirata Y, Kano H, Sato K, Watanabe Y, Watanabe TX, Nakajima K, Sakakibara S, and Marumo F. (1994) Specific receptors for adrenomedullin in cultured rat vascular smooth muscle cells. FEBS Lett 340:226-230.

Hagner S, Stahl U, Knoblauch B, McGregor GP, and Lang RE. (2002) Calcitonin receptor-like receptor: identification and distribution in human peripheral tissues. Cell Tissue Res 310:41-50.

Hamada H, Kitamura K, Chosa E, Eto T, and Tajima N. (2002) Adrenomedullin stimulates the growth of cultured normal human osteoblasts as an autocrine/paracrine regulator. Peptides 23:2163-2168.

Hinson JP, Kapas S, and Smith DM. (2000) Adrenomedullin, a multifunctional regulatory peptide. Endocr Rev 21:138-167.

Hirata Y, Hayakawa H, Suzuki Y, Suzuki E, Ikenouchi H, Kohmoto O, Kimura K, Kitamura K, Eto T, Kangawa K, Matsuo H, and Omata M. (1995) Mechanisms of adrenomedullin-induced vasodilation in the rat kidney. Hypertension 25:790-795.

Horio T, Kohno M, Kano H, Ikeda M, Yasunari K, Yokokawa K, Minami M, and Takeda T. (1995) Adrenomedullin as a novel antimigration factor of vascular smooth muscle cells. Circ Res 77:660-664.

Horio T, Nishikimi T, Yoshihara F, Matsuo H, Takishita S, and Kangawa K (1999) Effects of adrenomedullin on cultured rat cardiac myocytes and fibroblasts. Eur J Pharmacol 382:1-9.

Horio T, Nishikimi T, Yoshihara F, Nagaya N, Matsuo H, Takishita S, and Kangawa K. (1998) Production and secretion of adrenomedullin in cultured rat cardiac myocytes and nonmyocytes: stimulation by interleukin-1b and tumor necrosis factor-a. Endocrinology 139:4576-4580.

Ihara T, Ikeda U, Tate Y, Ishibashi S, and Shimada K. (2000) Positive inotropic effects of adrenomedullin on rat papillary muscle. Eur J Pharmacol

390:167-172.
Ikenouchi H, Kangawa K, Matsuo H, and Hirata Y. (1997) Negative inotropic effect of adrenomedullin in isolated adult rabbit cardiac ventricular myocytes. Circulation 95:2318-2324.
Ishiyama Y, Kitamura K, Ichiki Y, Nakamura S, Kida O, Kangawa K, and Eto T. (1993) Hemodynamic effects of a novel hypotensive peptide, human adrenomedullin, in rats. Eur J Pharmacol 241:271-273.
Isumi Y, Kubo A, Katafuchi T, Kangawa K, and Minamino N. (1999) Adrenomedullin suppresses interleukin-1b-induced tumor necrosis factor-a production in Swiss 3T3 cells. FEBS Lett 463:110-114.
Iwasaki H, Eguchi S, Shichiri M, Marumo F, and Hirata Y. (1998) Adrenomedullin as a novel growth-promoting factor for cultured vascular smooth muscle cells: role of tyrosine kinase-mediated mitogen-activated protein kinase activation. Endocrinology 139:3432-3441.
Jensen BL, Kramer BK, and Kurtz A. (1997) Adrenomedullin stimulates renin release and renin mRNA in mouse juxtaglomerular granular cells. Hypertension 29:1148-1155.
Jougasaki M, Aarhus LL, Heublein DM, Sandberg SM, and Burnett JC Jr. (1997) Role of prostaglandins and renal nerves in the renal actions of adrenomedullin. Am J Physiol 272:F260-F266.
Kamoi H, Kanazawa H, Hirata K, Kurihara N, Yano Y, and Otani S. (1995) Adrenomedullin inhibits the secretion of cytokine-induced neutrophil chemoattractant, a member of the interleukin-8 family, from rat alveolar macrophages. Biochem Biophys Res Commun 211:1031-1035.
Kanazawa H, Kurihara N, Hirata K, Kudoh S, Kawaguchi T, and Takeda T. (1994) Adrenomedullin, a newly discovered hypotensive peptide, is a potent bronchodilator. Biochem Biophys Res Commun 205:251-254.
Kano H, Kohno M, Yasunari K, Yokokawa K, Horio T, Ikeda M, Minami M, Hanehira T, Takeda T, and Yoshikawa J. (1996) Adrenomedullin as a novel antiproliferative factor of vascular smooth muscle cells. J Hypertens 14:209-213.
Kapas S, Martinez A, Cuttitta F, and Hinson JP (1998) Local production and action of adrenomedullin in the rat adrenal zona glomerulosa. J Endocrinol 156:477-484.
Kato H, Shichiri M, Marumo F, Hirata Y (1997) Adrenomedullin as an autocrine/paracrine apoptosis survival factor for rat endothelial cells. Endocrinology 138:2615-2620.
Kawada N and Inoue M. (1994) Effect of adrenomedullin on hepatic pericytes (stellate cells) of the rat. FEBS Lett 356:109-113.
Kawai J, Ando K, Tojo A, Shimosawa T, Takahashi K, Onozato ML, Yamasaki M, Ogita T, Nakaoka T, and Fujita T. (2004) Endogenous adrenomedullin protects against vascular response to injury in mice. Circulation 109:1147-

1153.
Kim W, Moon SO, Sung MJ, Kim SH, Lee S, So JN, and Park SK. (2003) Angiogenic role of adrenomedullin through activation of Akt, mitogen-activated protein kinase, and focal adhesion kinase in endothelial cells. FASEB J 17:1937-1939.
Kitamura K, Kangawa K, Kawamoto M, Ichiki Y, Nakamura S, Matsuo H, and Eto T. (1993) Adrenomedullin: a novel hypotensive peptide isolated from human pheochromocytoma. Biochem Biophys Res Commun 192:553-560.
Kohno M, Yokokawa K, Yasunari K, Kano H, Horio T, and Takeda T. (1995) Stimulation of cyclic adenosine monophosphate formation by the novel vasorelaxant peptide adrenomedullin in cultured rat mesangial cells. Metabolism 44:10-12.
Lai KN, Leung JC, Yeung VT, Lewis LK, and Nicholls MG. (1998) Gene transcription and synthesis of adrenomedullin by cultured human renal cells. Biochem Biophys Res Commun 244:567-572.
Lainchbury JG, Troughton RW, Lewis LK, Yandle TG, Richards AM, and Nicholls MG. (2000) Hemodynamic, hormonal, and renal effects of short-term adrenomedullin infusion in healthy volunteers. J Clin Endocrinol Metab 85:1016-1020.
Lang MG, Paterno R, Faraci FM, and Heistad DD. (1997) Mechanisms of adrenomedullin-induced dilatation of cerebral arterioles. Stroke 28:181-185.
Leclerc M and Brunette MG. (2000) The paradoxical effect of adrenomedullin on Na+ transport by the renal distal tubule luminal membrane. Mol Cell Endocrinol 164:159-167.
Lippton H, Chang JK, Hao Q, Summer W, and Hyman AL. (1994) Adrenomedullin dilates the pulmonary vascular bed *in vivo*. J Appl Physiol 76:2154-2156.
Lisy O, Jougasaki M, Schirger JA, Chen HH, Barclay PT, and Burnett JC Jr. (1998) Neutral endopeptidase inhibition potentiates the natriuretic actions of adrenomedullin. Am J Physiol 275:F410-F414.
Majid DS, Kadowitz PJ, Coy DH, and Navar LG. (1996) Renal responses to intra-arterial administration of adrenomedullin in dogs. Am J Physiol 270:F200-F205.
Malendowicz LK, Conconi MT, Parnigotto PP, and Nussdorfer GG. (2003) Endogenous adrenomedullin system regulates the growth of rat adrenocortical cells cultured in vitro. Regul Pept 112:27-31.
Marinoni E, Di Iorio R, Letizia C, Lucchini C, Alo P, and Cosmi EV. (2000) Changes in plasma adrenomedullin levels during the menstrual cycle. Regul Pept 87:15-18.
Marinoni E, Di Iorio R, Villaccio B, Letizia C, Aragona C, Schimberni M, and Cosmi EV. (2002) Follicular fluid adrenomedullin concentrations in

spontaneous and stimulated cycles: relationship to ovarian function and endothelin-1 and nitric oxide. Regul Pept 107:125-128.

Martinez A, Weaver C, Lopez J, Bhathena SJ, Elsasser TH, Miller MJ, Moody TW, Unsworth EJ, and Cuttitta F (1996) Regulation of insulin secretion and blood glucose metabolism by adrenomedullin. Endocrinology 137:2626-2632.

Martinez V, Cuttitta F, and Tache Y. (1997) Central action of adrenomedullin to inhibit gastric emptying in rats. Endocrinology 138:3749-3755.

Mazzocchi G, Albertin G, Andreis PG, Neri G, Malendowicz LK, Champion HC, Bahcelioglu M, Kadowitz PJ, and Nussdorfer GG. (1999) Distribution, functional role, and signaling mechanism of adrenomedullin receptors in the rat adrenal gland. Peptides 20:1479-1487.

McLatchie LM, Fraser NJ, Main MJ, Wise A, Brown J, Thompson N, Solari R, Lee MG, and Foord SM. (1998) RAMPs regulate the transport and ligand specificity of the calcitonin-receptor-like receptor. Nature 393:333-339.

Meeran K, O'Shea D, Upton PD, Small CJ, Ghatei MA, Byfield PH, and Bloom SR. (1997) Circulating adrenomedullin does not regulate systemic blood pressure but increases plasma prolactin after intravenous infusion in humans: a pharmacokinetic study. J Clin Endocrinol Metab 82:95-100.

Michibata H, Mukoyama M, Tanaka I, Suga S, Nakagawa M, Ishibashi R, Goto M, Akaji K, Fujiwara Y, Kiso Y, and Nakao K. (1998) Autocrine/paracrine role of adrenomedullin in cultured endothelial and mesangial cells. Kidney Int 53:979-985.

Miller MJ, Martinez A, Unsworth EJ, Thiele CJ, Moody TW, Elsasser T, and Cuttitta F. (1996) Adrenomedullin expression in human tumor cell lines. Its potential role as an autocrine growth factor. J Biol Chem 271:23345-51.

Miyashita K, Itoh H, Sawada N, Fukunaga Y, Sone M, Yamahara K, Yurugi-Kobayashi T, Park K, and Nakao K. (2003) Adrenomedullin provokes endothelial Akt activation and promotes vascular regeneration both in vitro and in vivo. FEBS Lett 544:86-92.

Montuenga LM, Martinez A, Miller MJ, Unsworth EJ, and Cuttitta F. (1997) Expression of adrenomedullin and its receptor during embryogenesis suggests autocrine or paracrine modes of action. Endocrinology 138:440-451.

Moriyama T, Otani T, and Maruo T. (2000) Expression of adrenomedullin by human granulosa lutein cells and its effect on progesterone production. Eur J Endocrinol 142:671-676.

Mulder H, Ahren B, Karlsson S, and Sundler F (1996) Adrenomedullin: localization in the gastrointestinal tract and effects on insulin secretion. Regul Pept 62:107-112.

Murphy TC and Samson WK. (1995) The novel vasoactive hormone, adrenomedullin, inhibits water drinking in the rat. Endocrinology

136:2459-2463.
Nagata D, Hirata Y, Suzuki E, Kakoki M, Hayakawa H, Goto A, Ishimitsu T, Minamino N, Ono Y, Kangawa K, Matsuo H, and Omata M. (1999) Hypoxia-induced adrenomedullin production in the kidney. Kidney Int 55:1259-1267.
Nagaya N, Nishikimi T, Horio T, Yoshihara F, Kanazawa A, Matsuo H, and Kangawa K. (1999) Cardiovascular and renal effects of adrenomedullin in rats with heart failure. Am J Physiol 276:R213-R218.
Nagaya N, Satoh T, Nishikimi T, Uematsu M, Furuichi S, Sakamaki F, Oya H, Kyotani S, Nakanishi N, Goto Y, Masuda Y, Miyatake K, and Kangawa K. (2000) Hemodynamic, renal, and hormonal effects of adrenomedullin infusion in patients with congestive heart failure. Circulation 101:498-503.
Nakamura Y, Shimatsu A, Murabe H, Mizuta H, Ihara C, and Nakao K. (1998) Calcitonin gene-related peptide as a GH secretagogue in human and rat pituitary somatotrophs. Brain Res 807:203-207.
Nishimatsu H, Suzuki E, Nagata D, Moriyama N, Satonaka H, Walsh K, Sata M, Kangawa K, Matsuo H, Goto A, Kitamura T, and Hirata Y. (2001) Adrenomedullin induces endothelium-dependent vasorelaxation *via* the phosphatidylinositol 3-kinase/Akt-dependent pathway in rat aorta. Circ Res 89:63-70.
Niu P, Shindo T, Iwata H, Iimuro S, Takeda N, Zhang Y, Ebihara A, Suematsu Y, Kangawa K, Hirata Y, and Nagai R. (2004) Protective Effects of Endogenous Adrenomedullin on Cardiac Hypertrophy, Fibrosis, and Renal Damage. Circulation (in press)
Nuki C, Kawasaki H, Kitamura K, Takenaga M, Kangawa K, Eto T, and Wada A. (1993) Vasodilator effect of adrenomedullin and calcitonin gene-related peptide receptors in rat mesenteric vascular beds. Biochem Biophys Res Commun 196:245-251.
Nussdorfer GG, Rossi GP, and Mazzocchi G (1997) Role of adrenomedullin and related peptides in the regulation of the hypothalamo-pituitary-adrenal axis. Peptides 18:1079-1089.
Osajima A, Mutoh Y, Uezono Y, Kawamura M, Izumi F, Takasugi M, and Kuroiwa A. (1995) Adrenomedullin increases cyclic AMP more potently than CGRP and amylin in rat renal tubular basolateral membranes. Life Sci 57:457-462.
Owada A, Nonoguchi H, Terada Y, Marumo F, and Tomita K. (1997) Microlocalization and effects of adrenomedullin in nephron segments and in mesangial cells of the rat. Am J Physiol 272:F691-F697.
Parameswaran N, Spielman WS, Pullen M, Francis J, Brooks DP, and Nambi P. (1999) Mechanism of adrenomedullin-stimulated hyaluronic acid release in rat mesangial cells. Eur J Pharmacol 370:313-318.
Parkes DG and May CN (1995) ACTH-suppressive and vasodilator actions of

adrenomedullin in conscious sheep. J Neuroendocrinol 7:923-929.

Petrie MC, Hillier C, Morton JJ, and McMurray JJ. (2000) Adrenomedullin selectively inhibits angiotensin II-induced aldosterone secretion in humans. J Hypertens 18:61-64.

Rossowski WJ, Jiang NY, and Coy DH. (1997) Adrenomedullin, amylin, calcitonin gene-related peptide and their fragments are potent inhibitors of gastric acid secretion in rats. Eur J Pharmacol 336:51-63.

Saita M, Shimokawa A, Kunitake T, Kato K, Hanamori T, Kitamura K, Eto T, and Kannan H. (1998) Central actions of adrenomedullin on cardiovascular parameters and sympathetic outflow in conscious rats. Am J Physiol 43:R979-R984.

Salomone S, Caruso A, Martinez G, Cutuli VM, Prato A, Bianchi A, Amico-Roxas M, and Clementi G. (2003) Secretory and vascular effects of adrenomedullin in gastric ulcer: role of CGRP- and adrenomedullin-receptors. Peptides 24:1175-1180.

Samson WK, Murphy T, and Schell DA (1995) A novel vasoactive peptide, adrenomedullin, inhibits pituitary adrenocorticotropin release. Endocrinology 136:2349-2352.

Serino R, Ueta Y, Hara Y, Nomura M, Yamamoto Y, Shibuya I, Hattori Y, Kitamura K, Kangawa K, Russell JA, and Yamashita H. (1999) Centrally administered adrenomedullin increases plasma oxytocin level with induction of c-fos messenger ribonucleic acid in the paraventricular and supraoptic nuclei of the rat. Endocrinology 140:2334-2342.

Shan J and Krukoff TL. (2001) Intracerebroventricular adrenomedullin stimulates the hypothalamic-pituitary-adrenal axis, the sympathetic nervous system and production of hypothalamic nitric oxide. J Neuroendocrinol 13:975-984.

Shimekake Y, Nagata K, Ohta S, Kambayashi Y, Teraoka H, Kitamura K, Eto T, Kangawa K, and Matsuo H. (1995) Adrenomedullin stimulates two signal transduction pathways, cAMP accumulation and Ca2+ mobilization, in bovine aortic endothelial cells. J Biol Chem 270:4412-4417.

Shimosawa T, Shibagaki Y, Ishibashi K, Kitamura K, Kangawa K, Kato S, Ando K, and Fujita T. (2002) Adrenomedullin, an endogenous peptide, counteracts cardiovascular damage. Circulation 105:106-111.

Stangl V, Dschietzig T, Bramlage P, Boye P, Kinkel HT, Staudt A, Baumann G, Felix SB, and Stangl K. (2000) Adrenomedullin and myocardial contractility in the rat. Eur J Pharmacol 408:83-89.

Szokodi I, Kinnunen P, Tavi P, Weckstrom M, Toth M, and Ruskoaho H. (1998) Evidence for cAMP-independent mechanisms mediating the effects of adrenomedullin, a new inotropic peptide. Circulation 97:1062-1070.

Takahashi H, Watanabe TX, Nishimura M, Nakanishi T, Sakamoto M, Yoshimura M, Komiyama Y, Masuda M, and Murakami T. (1994) Centrally induced vasopressor and sympathetic responses to a novel endogenous peptide, adrenomedullin, in anesthetized rats. Am J Hypertens 7:478-482.

Taniyama M, Kitamura K, Ban Y, Sugita E, Ito K, and Katagiri T. (1997) Elevation of circulating proadrenomedullin-N terminal 20-peptide in thyrotoxicosis. Clin Endocrinol (Oxf) 46:271-274.

Taylor GM, Meeran K, O'Shea D, Smith DM, Ghatei MA, and Bloom SR. (1996) Adrenomedullin inhibits feeding in the rat by a mechanism involving calcitonin gene-related peptide receptors. Endocrinology 137:3260-3264.

Tokudome T, Horio T, Yoshihara F, Suga S, Kawano Y, Kohno M, and Kangawa K. (2002) Adrenomedullin inhibits doxorubicin-induced cultured rat cardiac myocyte apoptosis via a cAMP-dependent mechanism. Endocrinology 143:3515-3521.

Tsuchida T, Ohnishi H, Tanaka Y, Mine T, and Fujita T. (1999) Inhibition of stimulated amylase secretion by adrenomedullin in rat pancreatic acini. Endocrinology 140:865-870.

Tsuruda T, Kato J, Kitamura K, Kuwasako K, Imamura T, Koiwaya Y, Tsuji T, Kangawa K, and Eto T. (1998) Adrenomedullin: a possible autocrine or paracrine inhibitor of hypertrophy of cardiomyocytes. Hypertension 31:505-510.

Wang X, Yue TL, Barone FC, White RF, Clark RK, Willette RN, Sulpizio AC, Aiyar NV, Ruffolo-RR J, and Feuerstein GZ. (1995) Discovery of adrenomedullin in rat ischemic cortex and evidence for its role in exacerbating focal brain ischemic damage. Proc Natl Acad Sci USA 92:11480-11484.

Wu R, Zhou M, and Wang P. (2003) Adrenomedullin and adrenomedullin binding protein-1 downregulate TNF-a in macrophage cell line and rat Kupffer cells. Regul Pept 112:19-26.

Yamaguchi T, Baba K, Doi Y, and Yano K (1995) Effect of adrenomedullin on aldosterone secretion by dispersed rat adrenal zona glomerulosa cells. Life Sci 56:379-387.

Yamaguchi T, Baba K, Doi Y, Yano K, Kitamura K, and Eto T (1996) Inhibition of aldosterone production by adrenomedullin, a hypotensive peptide, in the rat. Hypertension 28:308-314.

Yanagita T, Yamamoto R, Sugano T, Kobayashi H, Uezono Y, Yokoo H, Shiraishi S, Minami SI, and Wada A. (2000) Adrenomedullin inhibits spontaneous and bradykinin-induced but not oxytocin- or prostaglandin F_{2a}-induced periodic contraction of rat uterus. Br J Pharmacol 130:1727-1730.

Yin H, Chao L, and Chao J. (2004) Adrenomedullin protects against myocardial apoptosis after ischemia/reperfusion through activation of Akt-GSK signaling. Hypertension 43:109-116.

Yokoi H, Arima H, Murase T, Kondo K, Iwasaki Y, and Oiso Y. (1996) Intracerebroventricular injection of adrenomedullin inhibits vasopressin

release in conscious rats. Neurosci Lett 216:65-67.
Yoshihara F, Horio T, Nishikimi T, Matsuo H, and Kangawa K. (2002) Possible involvement of oxidative stress in hypoxia-induced adrenomedullin secretion in cultured rat cardiomyocytes. Eur J Pharmacol 436:1-6.
Yoshihara F, Nishikimi T, Okano I, Horio T, Yutani C, Matsuo H, Takishita S, Ohe T, and Kangawa K. (2001) Alterations of intrarenal adrenomedullin and its receptor system in heart failure rats. Hypertension 37:216-222.
Yoshimoto R, MitsuiSaito M, Ozaki H, and Karaki H. (1998) Effects of adrenomedullin and calcitonin gene-related peptide on contractions of the rat aorta and porcine coronary artery. Br J Pharmacol 123:1645-1654.
Zhao Y, Hague S, Manek S, Zhang L, Bicknell R, and Rees MCP. (1998) PCR display identifies tamoxifen induction of the novel angiogenic factor adrenomedullin by a non estrogenic mechanism in the human endometrium. Oncogene 16:409-415.
Ziolkowska A, Budzynska K, Trejter M, Tortorella C, Belloni AS, and Malendowicz LK. (2003) Effects of adrenomedullin and its fragment 22-52 on basal and ACTH-stimulated secretion of cultured rat adrenocortical cells. Int J Mol Med 11:613-615.
Zudaire E, Cuttitta F, and Martinez A. (2003a) Regulation of pancreatic physiology by adrenomedullin and its binding protein. Regul Pept 112:121-130.
Zudaire E, Martinez A, and Cuttitta F. (2003b) Adrenomedullin and cancer. Regul Pept 112:175-183.

6

CIRCULATING ADRENOMEDULLIN

Toshio Nishikimi

Department of Hypertension and Cardiorenal Medicine, Dokkyo University School of Medicine, Mibu, Tochigi 321-0293, Japan

1. ADRENOMEDULLIN ASSAYS

In the first report about adrenomedullin (AM) by Kitamura et al (Kitamura et al., 1993a), plasma AM levels were measured by radioimmunoassay after digestion with trypsin. It was found that plasma AM levels in humans were 19 fmol/mL. The same group developed a simpler radioimmunoassay system after extraction of plasma (Kitamura et al.,1994). In that report, plasma levels of AM were 3.3 fmol/mL. Other investigators also developed their own radioimmunoassay systems using polyclonal antibodies and reported that the plasma levels of AM were 3 - 8 fmol/mL. In general, these assay systems reported in the literature appear to have been carefully validated, with evidence presented from high performance liquid chromatography analysis to show that immunoreactive AM from human plasma coelutes with authentic human AM (Kohno et al.,1996; Lewis et al., 1998). Therefore, the absolute plasma levels of AM in the normal human appear to be consistent. Various studies have shown that the plasma levels of AM in the normal human are 1 - 10 fmol/mL. In general, they revealed that sex or age does not affect the plasma AM levels. However, recent observations showed that plasma AM levels increase in association with aging in the normal human, especially in humans over 70 years old (Kato et al., 2002). No circadian variation of plasma AM levels was found in normal humans (Nishikimi et al., 2001).

2. ORIGIN AND METABOLIC SITES OF ADRENOMEDULLIN

(1) Origin of circulating adrenomedullin

AM was initially discovered in human pheochromocytoma by monitoring the cAMP activity in rat platelets (Kitamura et al.,1993a). AM mRNA is highly expressed not only in pheochromocytoma but also in normal adrenal medulla, kidney, lungs, and ventricle (Kitamura et al., 1993b). However, whether these organs secrete AM into circulation or not was not initially fully understood. To investigate the sites of production and clearance of AM in humans, we took samples of both arterial and venous blood across the adrenal gland, kidney, lung, and heart and measured plasma AM concentrations by radioimmunoassay (Nishikimi et al., 1994). There was no step-up of plasma AM concentration in the coronary sinus, renal vein, or adrenal vein. There were no significant differences in plasma AM concentrations among the various sites of the right side of the heart including the inferior portion of the inferior vena cava, superior portion of the inferior vena cava, superior vena cava, right atrium, right ventricle, and pulmonary artery. Plasma AM levels in the aorta were slightly but significantly lower than those in pulmonary artery. Furthermore, in a patient with a pheochromocytoma, no change in plasma AM concentration was seen during a hypertensive attack, although both epinephrine and norepinephrine concentrations increased markedly (Nishikimi et al., 1994). Subsequent studies supported the notion that the AM level in the adrenal vein was not increased and does not contribute to the main source of plasma AM (Kato et al., 1995; Minami et al., 2002). Although it has been shown that AM is cosecreted with catecholamines, at least by bovine chromaffin cells in culture (Katoh et al., 1994), these data suggest that the adrenal medulla is unlikely to be a significant source of circulating AM. Thus, although AM peptide and mRNA expression are widely distributed in various tissues and organs, the main source of plasma AM in vivo is now thought to be the vasculature, because AM mRNA is more prominently expressed in vascular endothelial cells and smooth muscle cells than in the adrenal gland (Sugo et al., 1994a; Sugo et al., 1994b). This hypothesis is consistent with the results described above.

(2) Metabolic clearance of adrenomedullin

The plasma half-life of AM has been reported to be 22.0 ± 1.6 min with an metabolic clearance rate of 27.4 ± 3.6 ml/kg/min and with an apparent volume of distribution of 880 ± 150 ml/kg (Meeran et al., 1997). The effects of plasma membrane enzymes on AM have been investigated. It appears likely that AM is degraded initially by metalloproteases to yield AM 8-52, 26-52, and 33-52, followed by an aminopeptidase action to yield AM 2-52, 27-52, and 28-52 (Lewis et al., 1997). We also reported that the lung is a major site of AM clearance in man (Nishikimi et al., 1994). Furthermore, we reported that active mature AM (AM-m), a 52 amino acid peptide with a C-terminal amide structure, is specifically extracted in the pulmonary circulation (Nishikimi et al., 2001; Nishikimi et al., 2002). Neutral endopeptidase is localized in greatest abundance in the kidney and cleaves endogenous peptides like AM, which possesses a disulfide ring. Lisy et al. (Lisy et al., 1998) reported that neutral endopeptidase inhibition potentiates the natriuretic actions of exogenous AM in anesthetized dogs, suggesting that AM is also degraded by the neutral endopeptidase.

3. MATURE AND GLYCINE-EXTENDED AM

AM is produced from AM precursor by the two steps of enzymatic reaction. First, AM precursor consisting of 185 amino acids is converted to glycine-extended AM (AM-Gly), a 53-amino acid peptide that is an inactive intermediate form of AM. Subsequently, AM-Gly is converted to active mature AM (AM-m), a 52-amino acid peptide with a C-terminal amide structure, by enzymatic amidation (Figure 1). Kitamura et al. (Kitamura et al., 1998) reported that two molecular forms of AM, AM-m and AM-Gly, circulate in human blood and that the major molecular form in human plasma is AM-Gly. They measured the levels of two molecular forms of AM, using two kinds of radioimmunoassay systems after the extraction of large amounts of plasma.

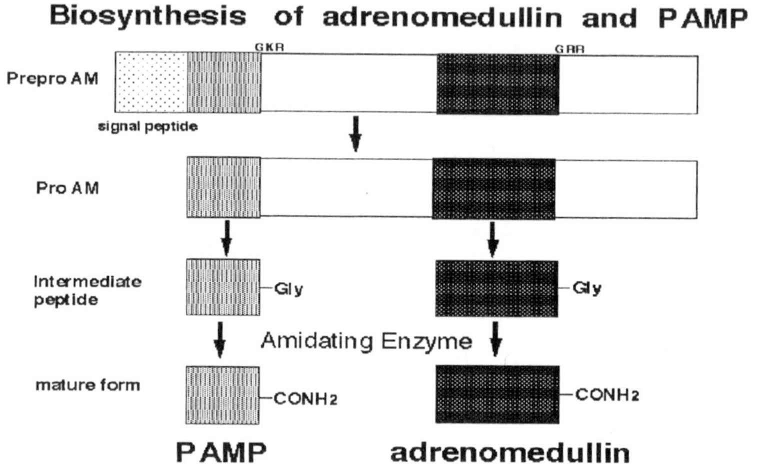

Figure 1. Biosynthesis of adrenomedullin (AM) is shown. AM and proadrenomedullin N-terminal 20 peptide (PAMP) are synthesized from the same AM precursor (prepro AM). Prepro AM (185 amino acids) is first converted to glycine-extended AM (AM-Gly), a 53-amino-acid peptide that is an inactive intermediate form of AM. Then, AM-Gly is converted to active mature AM (AM-m), a 52-amino-acid peptide with a C-terminal amide structure ($CONH_2$), by enzymatic amidation. AM-T = (AM-m) + (AM-Gly).

Ohta et al. (Ohta et al., 1999a, Ohta et al., 1999b) developed new immunoradiometric assay kits for the measurement of both AM-m and AM-T (AM-T = AM-m + AM-Gly) (AM mature RIA SHIONOGI, AM RIA SHIONOGI, Shionogi Pharmaceutical Co., Ltd., Osaka, Japan). These assay systems use two monoclonal antibodies against human AM, one recognizing the ring structure of human AM in both kits and the other recognizing the carboxy-terminal sequence in the AM-m kit or AM (25-36) in the AM-T kit. The assay measures human AM-m or AM-T by sandwiching it between the two antibodies without the extraction of plasma. A reverse-phase high-performance liquid chromatography analysis revealed that the major peak of immunoreactive AM in the plasma detected by each immunoradiometric assay kit for AM-m and AM-T was identical to synthetic human AM (1-52). Using this kit we and other investigators reported that plasma AM-T levels in normal human plasma are about 10 fmol/mL (Ohta et al., 1999a, Nishikimi et al., 2000).

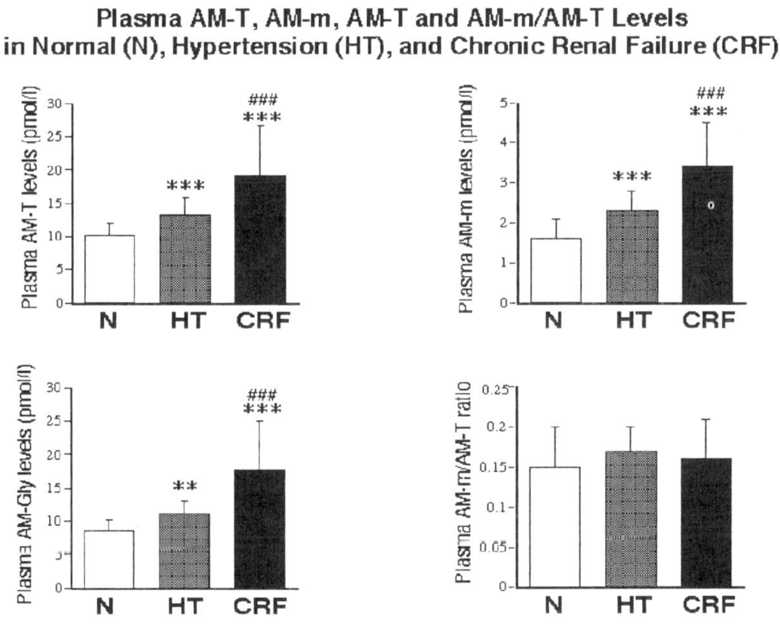

Figure 2. Plasma AM-T, AM-m, AM-Gly and AM-m/AM-T ratio in normal controls (N), and in patients with essential hypertension (HT) and chronic renal failure (CRF). ** $P < 0.01$ vs N, *** $P < 0.001$ vs N, ### $P < 0.001$ vs HT

In hypertension, renal failure, congestive heart failure, acute myocardial infarction and pulmonary hypertension, both plasma AM-Gly and AM-m levels are increased and the ratio of AM-Gly to AM-m does not significantly change (Figure 2). (Nishikimi et al., 2001a; Asakawa et al., 2001; Nishikimi et al., 2001b).

We measured two molecular forms of AM in rat tissue and plasma using this system. We found that the major molecular form in plasma is AM-Gly, as observed in human plasma (Tadokoro et al., 2003). However, the major molecular form of AM is AM-m in left ventricular tissue in normotensive and hypertensive rats, and the AM-m/AM-T ratio is further increased in severe left ventricular hypertrophy (Nishikimi et al., 2003; Wang et al., 2003).

4. PLASAM AM LEVELS IN CARDIOVASCULAR DISEASES

(1) Plasma AM levels in hypertension

Regarding the physiological action of AM, it is suggested that AM is involved in the pathophysiology of hypertension.

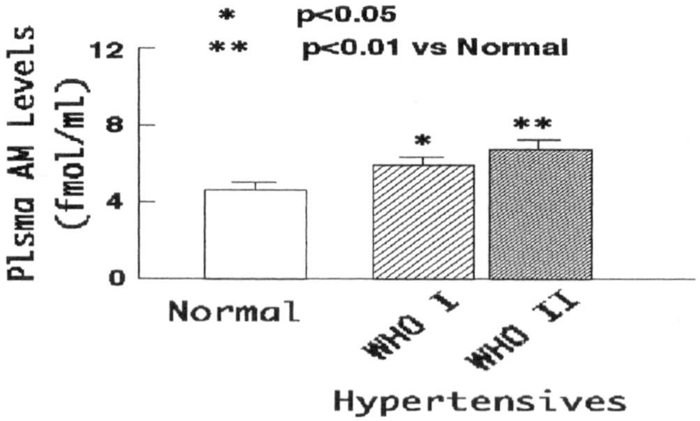

Figure 3. Plasma AM levels in normal subjects, essential hypertensive subjects with WHO stage I, and essential hypertensive subjects with WHO stage II.

Ishimitsu et al. (Ishimitsu et al., 1994) first reported that plasma AM is increased in hypertensive patients with WHO stage I compared to normal subjects and further increased in hypertensive patients with WHO stage II (Figure 3). Plasma levels of AM are correlated with hypertensive organ damage, suggesting that increased plasma AM may reflect an overflow from local sites of production. Indeed, Shimokubo et al. reported that in rat hypertension model left ventricular tissue AM levels are correlated with plasma AM levels, suggesting that AM may be produced and secreted in the hypertrophied heart (Shimokubo et al., 1996). Sumimoto et al. (Sumimoto et al., 1997) also reported that plasma AM levels are higher in patients with left ventricular hypertrophy than in those without it and that plasma AM levels are correlated with left ventricular mass index. In the experimental model of left ventricular hypertrophy, mRNA and tissue levels of AM in the left ventricle are increased and are considered to partly contribute to the plasma levels of AM (Morimoto et al., 1999). However, this contribution is not so large compared with the large contribution of systemic vascular bed. Kohno et al. (Kohno et al., 1996) reported that plasma AM levels are correlated with creatinine clearance. Although it is a fact that plasma AM levels are correlated with the degree of renal dysfunction, whether increased AM levels are explained not only by the decrease of creatinine clearance, but also by increased plasma volume remains unclear. Because plasma AM levels in the renal vein are higher than those in the renal artery, AM may be produced rather than consumed in the kidney (Nishikimi et al., 1994; Nishikimi et al., 2000). In malignant hypertension, plasma AM levels are markedly increased compared with those in essential hypertension and their increase is reduced after adequate antihypertensive treatment (Nishikimi et al., 1996; Kato et al., 1999). In addition, it is reported that plasma AM levels are increased in patients with primary aldosteronism (Kato et al., 1995). Taken together, these results indicate that plasma AM levels are increased in proportion to the disease severity in hypertension and that increased AM may function in a defense mechanism. Thus, it appears reasonable to speculate that elevated AM is a consequence rather than a cause of the pathology.

Regarding the molecular form of AM, Kitamura et al. first reported that AM-Gly and AM-m are similarly elevated in essential hypertensive subjects (Kitamura et al., 1998). Using two kinds of radioimmunoassay which recognize the entire AM molecule and C-terminal amide structure, they characterized human plasma AM immunoreactivity chromatographically. Using gel filtration and reverse phase high-performance liquid chromatography analyses, they showed that most of the AM immunoreactivity measured by a radioimmunoassay which recognized the entire AM molecule was eluted at a position identical to where AM-Gly eluted and was not recognized by a radioimmunoassay which recognized the C-terminal amide structure. They concluded that most circulating plasma AM immunoreactivity consists of AM-Gly, an intermediate form of AM.

In addition, we also measured plasma and urinary AM levels in patients with hypertension and chronic renal failure (Nishikimi et al., 2001a). Plasma AM-m, AM-Gly and AM-T levels were increased in patients with hypertension and chronic renal failure compared with normal subjects, whereas urinary AM-m, AM-Gly and AM-T excretions were decreased in patients with hypertension and chronic renal failure compared with normal subjects. Urinary AM-m/AM-T ratios were significantly higher than plasma AM-m/AM-T ratios. Taken together, these results suggest that plasma AM-m in parallel with AM-Gly is increased in hypertension and chronic renal failure; urine contains a higher percentage of active AM than plasma; and urinary AM levels are decreased in patients with hypertension and chronic renal failure compared with normal subjects. The origin of AM in plasma and urine may be different; it has been suggested that the origin of plasma is the vasculature. In contrast, urinary AM may be derived from renal tubular cells rather than from plasma because an autoradiographic study using venous injection of ^{125}I-AM revealed that intense ^{125}I-AM uptake was observed in the proximal tubules, suggesting that most plasma AM filtered by the glomerulus is reabsorbed by the proximal tubular cells (Hasegawa et al., 1998). Thus, the decrease in urinary AM excretion in chronic renal failure may in part be explained by the decreased number of nephrons producing AM.

A variety of evidence has been accumulated regarding the role of increased AM in hypertension. An intravenous injection of rat AM dose-dependently reduced the mean blood pressure with a concomitant fall in total peripheral resistance index and an increase in cardiac index in normotensive and hypertensive rats (Ishiyama et al., 1995). Khan et al (Khan et al., 1997) reported the chronic effect of AM infusion on the blood pressure in hypertensive rats. They showed that chronically infused human AM has a hypotensive effect in normotensive and hypertensive rats at plasma AM concentration within the physiological range. They also investigated the effect of chronic AM infusion in rats with renovascular hypertension (Khan et al., 1997). They showed that AM reduces blood pressure, plasma renin activity, and aldosterone concentrations at plasma AM concentrations within the physiological range. Thus, not only a hypotensive effect, but also an inhibitory effect on the renin-aldosterone system by AM, was suggested. We also reported the effects of chronic infusion of human AM in severe hypertensive rats (Nishikimi et al., 2002; Mori et al, 2002). Chronic AM treatment significantly improved renal function and histological findings without changing mean arterial pressure. Interestingly, long-term human AM infusion decreased the endogenous rat AM level with a slight increase of human AM level. Chronic AM treatment also significantly inhibited the increases of plasma renin concentration, aldosterone level, and renal tissue angiotensin II level. Furthermore, AM infusion significantly attenuated the increases of mRNA expression of TGF-beta and angiotensin-converting enzyme in the renal cortex. These results suggest that increased endogenous AM plays a compensatory role in chronic hypertensive renal failure and that long-term AM infusion has renoprotective effects in this type of hypertension model, partly via inhibition of the circulating and renal renin-angiotensin system. We also analyzed the effect of chronic AM infusion on the transition from left ventricular hypertrophy to heart failure (Nishikimi et al., 2003). Chronic AM infusion significantly improved hemodynamics and left ventricular weight/body weight. In addition, AM significantly attenuated the increases in circulating renin-aldosterone, endogenous rat AM, and atrial natriuretic peptide (ANP) levels. AM also decreased the myocardial tissue levels of angiotensin II and atrial and brain natriuretic peptide (BNP). These changes were associated with the improvement of cardiac output, systemic vascular resistance, and left ventricular end-systolic elastance. These results suggest that endogenous AM plays a compensatory role in heart failure and that chronic AM infusion attenuates the transition from left ventricular hypertrophy to heart failure at least in part through inhibition of circulating and myocardial neurohormonal activation. In addition, Dobrzynski et al. (Dobrzynski, et al., 2000) reported the effects of AM gene delivery in deoxycorticosterone acetate-salt hypertensive rats. Human AM gene delivery resulted in a prolonged reduction of blood pressure and improved renal function. Human AM gene delivery significantly reduced glomerular sclerosis, tubular injury, luminol protein cast accumulation, and interstitial fibrosis as well as urinary protein in the kidney. In the heart, human AM gene delivery caused significant decreases in left ventricular weight and cardiomyocyte diameter, which were accompanied by reduced interstitial fibrosis and extracellular matrix formation within the heart. Thus, it is possible that increased AM in hypertension may function in a protective mechanism.

(2) Plasma AM Levels in Heart Failure

There have been several reports which showed that plasma AM levels are increased in heart failure in proportion to the disease severity (Nishikimi et al., 1995; Jougasaki et al., 1995, Kato et al., 1996). We showed that there was no increase of plasma AM level in patients with NYHA class I; however, plasma AM levels slightly but significantly increased in patients with NYHA class II. Furthermore, they were further increased in NYHA class III or IV (Figure 4). Plasma AM levels were positively correlated with the plasma ANP, BNP and norepinephrine levels and negatively correlated with left ventricular ejection fraction (Nishikimi et al., 1995)..

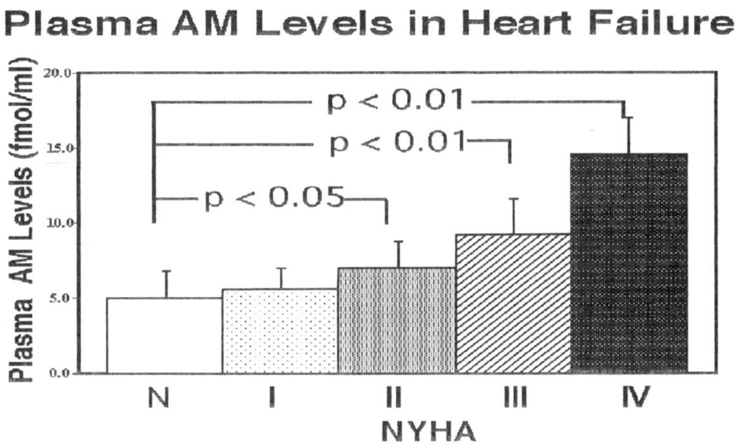

Figure 4. Plasma levels of adrenomedullin (AM) in patients with heart failure in NYHA functional classes I, II, III, and IV and normal subjects (N).

After the treatment of heart failure, plasma ANP and BNP rapidly decreased, whereas the plasma AM level decreased relatively slowly (Nishikimi et al., 1995). These results indicate that plasma AM levels are increased in proportion to the severity of the disease and that the mechanism of their increase may be related to the increased plasma volume and/or sympathetic nerve activity. This finding is consistent with an other report which showed a good relationship between plasma AM levels and pulmonary capillary wedge pressure (Kobayashi et al., 1996a).

On the other hand, recent studies revealed that two molecular forms of AM circulate in human plasma and that the major circulating form is an inactive form, AM-Gly (Kitamura et al., 1998; Nishikimi et al., 2000). Hirayama et al. reported that both molecular forms of AM are similarly increased in patients with heart failure (Hirayama et al., 1999). Thus, AM may respond to the pathophysiology of heart failure and may be a biochemical marker for the severity of heart failure. Recent reports which showed that plasma AM level is an independent prognostic indicator of mild to moderate heart failure (Pousset et al., 2000) and ischemic heart failure with left ventricular dysfunction (Richards et al., 2001) support this hypothesis. Thus, AM may be not only an important biochemical marker for evaluating the severity of heart failure, but also a prognostic indicator of this syndrome. Thus, AM may be included in the routine clinical workup of patients with heart failure.

(3) Plasma AM levels in acute myocardial infarction

Kobayashi et al. (Kobayashi et al., 1996b) first reported that plasma AM was higher immediately after the onset of AMI and decreased gradually. They showed that plasma AM levels were higher in patients with congestive heart failure than in patients without congestive heart failure throughout the period of the study. They showed that plasma AM was positively correlated with pulmonary capillary wedge pressure, pulmonary arterial pressure, right atrial pressure, and heart rate in the early stage of AMI. Miyao et al. (Miyao et al., 1998) also serially measured plasma levels of AM in 31 patients with acute myocardial infarction over 4 weeks. In patients with acute myocardial infarction, plasma AM levels reached a peak at 24 hours after the onset of symptoms and remained increased at all sampling points except the four-week point compared with the value in normal subjects (Figure 5). AM concentrations on admission were higher in patients from Killip classes II, III, and IV than class I, and were correlated positively with peak plasma creatine kinase and left ventricular end diastolic volume index, and negatively with left ventricular ejection fraction. The values from 12 to 48 hours were negatively correlated with systemic vascular resistance index.

During the time course studied, AM concentrations were positively correlated with ANP and BNP. They concluded that plasma AM concentrations increased in the acute phase of myocardial infarction in proportion with clinical severity. Yoshitomi et al. (Yoshitomi et al., 1998) also reported that plasma AM levels on admission were correlated with ANP levels. They showed that success of reperfusion by percutaneous transluminal coronary angioplasty did not affect the plasma AM level. They speculated that volume expansion might be one of the additional stimuli for the release of AM in patients with acute myocardial infarction complicated by congestive heart failure.

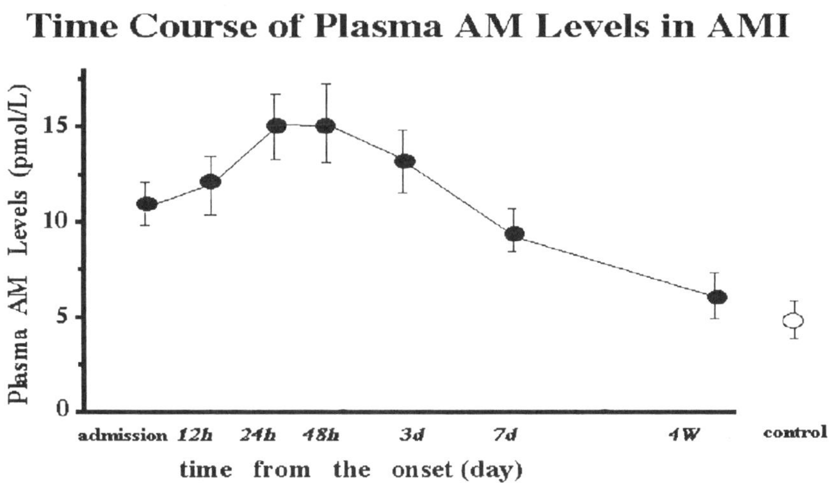

Figure 5. Time course of plasma AM levels in patients with acute myocardial infarction.

In addition, we examined whether prognosis after acute myocardial infarction can be predicted by measuring plasma AM levels (Nagaya et al., 1999). Plasma AM concentrations on day 2 after myocardial infarction were measured in 113 patients with myocardial infarction with other clinical and haemodynamic variables related to mortality. During a mean follow up period of 25 months, 16 patients died of cardiac causes. Plasma AM was correlated negatively with left ventricular ejection fraction on admission. By univariate Cox proportional hazards analysis, plasma AM, age, coronary reperfusion, maximum creatine kinase concentrations, pulmonary congestion, pulmonary capillary wedge pressure, cardiac index, and left ventricular ejection fraction were all significantly related to mortality. Among the non-invasive variables, only plasma AM was an independent predictor of mortality after myocardial infarction. The Kaplan-Meier survival curves based on the median plasma AM concentration showed that patients with high plasma AM had a higher mortality than those with low plasma AM. Richard et al. (Richard et al., 1998) compared several neurohumoral factors as prognostic markers after acute myocardial infarction. They showed that plasma AM levels have a significant inverse relation with LV function, which is comparable to that of norepinephrine. They also showed that plasma AM is predictive of death in the 2 years after myocardial infarction, but this relation is generally weaker than observed for N-terminal proBNP (N-BNP). As a reason for the weaker prognostic value of AM compared with that of N-BNP, they speculated that increased plasma AM levels in heart failure are mediated by a variety of mechanisms, including induction of endothelial production of AM, elevated levels of endothelin, or other humoral and neural mechanisms. Hence AM appears to be an indirect reflector of LV function and has a weaker association with LV size or contractile function or prognosis than BNP or N-BNP.

Regarding the molecular forms of AM in acute myocardial infarction, Asakawa et al. (Asakawa et al., 2001) investigated the pathophysiological significance of the two molecular forms of AM in plasma and urine in patients with acute myocardial infarction. Plasma AM-m, AM-Gly and AM-T levels were increased on admission in patients with acute myocardial infarction and reached a peak 24 h after the onset of symptoms. Plasma AM-m, AM-Gly and AM-T levels were significantly correlated with plasma levels of BNP and pulmonary arterial pressure. In contrast, urinary excretion of AM-m, AM-Gly and AM-T was also increased on admission, and reached a peak at 12 h after the onset of symptoms. Urinary excretion of AM-m and AM-Gly was significantly correlated with urinary sodium excretion. AM-m levels were significantly correlated with AM-Gly levels in both the urine and plasma; however, there were no significant correlations between plasma and urinary AM levels. The results suggest that the levels of both molecular forms of AM are increased in the urine as well as in the plasma in the acute myocardial infarction. They speculated that increased concentrations of AM in plasma and urine in the acute myocardial infarction may be involved in the mechanism of defense against further elevations of peripheral and pulmonary vascular resistance and oliguria in acute myocardial infarction.

To date, the pathophysiological role of the upregulation of AM in AMI is not fully understood. Previous studies have demonstrated that AM is an antihypertrophic peptide able to inhibit hypertrophy induced by angiotensin II or endothelin-1 in cultured neonatal cardiac myocytes and fibroblasts (Tsuruda et al., 1998; Tsuruda et al., 1999). In addition, AM significantly attenuates the collagen production and proliferation of cardiac fibroblasts, possibly via a cAMP-dependent mechanism (Horio et al., 1999). These findings suggest a possible role of AM as an antiremodeling autocrine and/or paracrine factor in the heart. Indeed, recent studies demonstrated that continuous administration of AM has beneficial effects on left ventricular remodeling and hemodynamics in AMI *in vivo* (Nakamura et al., 2002). In addition, AM is reported to exert a direct inotropic effect in vitro and to increase myocardial contractility in vivo (Szokodi et al., 1998). In fact, intravenous administration of AM enhanced left ventricular myocardial contraction and improved left ventricular relaxation without increasing myocardial oxygen consumption in patients with left ventricular dysfunction (Nagaya et al., 2002). These results suggest that increased cardiac production of AM-m may compensate LV dysfunction caused by AMI. Furthermore, a recent study showed that AM significantly attenuated myocardial ischemia/reperfusion injury via a PI3K/Akt-dependent pathway

(Okumura et al., 2004). Other investigators also showed that delivery of the AM gene protects against cardiomyocyte apoptosis induced by ischemia/reperfusion injury through the Akt-GSK-caspase signaling pathway (Yin et al., 2004). Taken together, these results suggest that increased mature-type AM in the heart may exert a cardioprotective effect in patients with LV dysfunction.

(4) Plasma AM levels in pulmonary hypertension

In pulmonary hypertension, Yoshibayashi et al. (Yoshibayashi et al., 1997) showed that plasma AM levels were significantly elevated in young patients with pulmonary hypertension and that there were significant differences in the plasma AM levels in the pulmonary artery and vein, suggesting a role of AM in pulmonary circulation. We also showed (Nishikimi et al., 1997) that plasma concentrations of AM are elevated in secondary pulmonary hypertension due to mitral stenosis and that they are correlated with mean pulmonary artery pressure, total pulmonary vascular resistance, and pulmonary vascular resistance. Kakishita et al. (Kakishita et al., 1999) reported that plasma levels of AM were significantly higher in patients with pulmonary hypertension than in control subjects, and that plasma levels of AM were significantly correlated with mean right atrial pressure, stroke volume, total pulmonary resistance, mean pulmonary arterial pressure, and the plasma ANP. These results suggest that plasma levels of AM increase in proportion to the extent of pulmonary hypertension and that plasma AM was partially extracted in the pulmonary circulation despite of the different etiology.

Regarding the molecular type of AM, we showed (Nishikimi et al., 2001) that AM-m, but not AM-Gly is extracted in the lung, suggesting that extracted AM-m in the lungs may help to attenuate the increased pulmonary arterial resistance. Furthermore, in a study of the effect of AM on the hemodynamics and hormonal response, Nagaya et al. (Nagaya et al., 2000) demonstrated that the intravenous infusion of AM (0.05 microgram/kg/min) produced a 44% increase in cardiac index and a 32% decrease in pulmonary vascular resistance, with a 4% reduction in mean pulmonary arterial pressure together with a reduction of the plasma aldosterone level. Taken together, these results indicate that increased plasma AM levels in the pulmonary circulation may be involved in defense mechanisms by causing dilation of pulmonary vessels and increased pulmonary blood flow.

(5) Plasma AM levels in congenital heart disease

Yoshibayashi et al. (Yoshibayashi et al., 1997) first reported that plasma AM concentrations are elevated in younger patients with congenital heart disease. They showed that plasma AM concentrations in congenital cyanotic heart disease were significantly (3-fold) higher than those in normal subjects. They compared plasma AM levels between the pulmonary artery and pulmonary vein and found that plasma AM concentrations in pulmonary venous blood were significantly lower than those in pulmonary arterial blood, again suggesting the extraction of plasma AM in the pulmonary circulation. Watanabe et al. (Watanabe et al., 2003) measured AM-m and AM-Gly in young patients with congenital heart disease and found that each molecular form of AM was negatively correlated with mixed venous oxygen saturation and systemic arterial oxygen saturation, and positively correlated with pulmonary arterial resistance, suggesting that hypoxia is an important stimulus for AM secretion. They showed that the venous AM-m level was significantly higher than the arterial AM-m, suggesting that the mature form is extracted in the pulmonary circulation, whereas there were no venoarterial differences in AM-Gly.

In summary, plasma AM levels are increased in various cardiovascular diseases in proportion to the disease severity. Elevated AM may be a consequence rather than a cause of the pathology. It is possible that systemic increases in AM reflect an overflow from local sites of production and that increased AM has both local and systemic compensatory roles in various cardiovascular diseases.

REFERENCES

Asakawa H, Nishikimi T, Suzuki T, Hara S, Tsubokou Y, Yagi H, Yabe A, Tsuchiya N, Horinaka S, Kangawa K, Matsuoka H. (2001) Elevation of two molecular forms of adrenomedullin in plasma and urine in patients with acute myocardial infarction treated with early coronary angioplasty. Clin Sci. 100:117-126.

Dobrzynski E, Wang C, Chao J, Chao L. (2000) Adrenomedullin gene delivery attenuates hypertension, cardiac remodeling, and renal injury in deoxycorticosterone acetate-salt hypertensive rats. Hypertension. 36:995-1001.

Hasegawa H, Mizuhira V, Notoya M, Inazawa K, Mizojiri K, Kitamura K, Kangawa K. (1998) Autoradiographic studies on the binding sites of 125I-adrenomedullin in rat tissues. Acta Histochem Cytochem 31:335-343

Hirayama N, Kitamura K, Imamura T, Kato J, Koiwaya Y, Tsuji T, Kangawa K, Eto T. (1999) Molecular forms of circulating adrenomedullin in patients with congestive heart failure. J Endocrinol. 160:297-303.

Horio T, Nishikimi T, Yoshihara F, Matsuo H, Takishita S, Kangawa K. (1999) Effects of adrenomedullin on cultured rat cardiac myocytes and fibroblasts. Eur J Pharmacol. 382:1-9.

Ishimitsu T, Nishikimi T, Saito Y, Kitamura K, Eto T, Kangawa K, Matsuo H, Omae T, Matsuoka H. (1994) Plasma levels of adrenomedullin, a newly identified hypotensive peptide, in patients with hypertension and renal failure. J Clin Invest. 94:2158-2161.

Ishiyama Y, Kitamura K, Ichiki Y, Nakamura S, Kida O, Kangawa K, Eto T. (1993) Hemodynamic effects of a novel hypotensive peptide, human adrenomedullin, in rats. Eur J Pharmacol. 241:271-273.

Jougasaki M, Wei CM, McKinley LJ, Burnett JC Jr. (1995) Elevation of circulating and ventricular adrenomedullin in human congestive heart failure. Circulation. 92:286-289.

Kakishita M, Nishikimi T, Okano Y, Satoh T, Kyotani S, Nagaya N, Fukushima K, Nakanishi N, Takishita S, Miyata A, Kangawa K, Matsuo H, Kunieda T. (1999) Increased plasma levels of adrenomedullin in patients with pulmonary hypertension. Clin Sci. 96:33-39.

Kato J, Kobayashi K, Etoh T, Tanaka M, Kitamura K, Imamura T, Koiwaya Y, Kangawa K, Eto T. (1996) Plasma adrenomedullin concentration in patients with heart failure. J Clin Endocrinol Metab. 81:180-183.

Kato J, Kitamura K, Matsui E, Tanaka M, Ishizaka Y, Kita T, Kangawa K, Eto T. (1999) Plasma adrenomedullin and natriuretic peptides in patients with essential or malignant hypertension. Hypertens Res. 22:61-65.

Kato J, Kitamura K, Uemura T, Kuwasako K, Kita T, Kangawa K, Eto T. (2002) Plasma levels of adrenomedullin and atrial and brain natriuretic peptides in the general population: their relations to age and pulse pressure. Hypertens Res. 25:887-892.

Katoh F, Niina H, Kitamura K, Ichiki Y, Yamamoto Y, Kangawa K, Eto T, Wada A. (1994) $Ca^{(2+)}$-dependent cosecretion of adrenomedullin and catecholamines mediated by nicotinic receptors in bovine cultured adrenal medullary cells. FEBS Lett.348:61-64.

Kato K, Kitamura K, Kuwasako K, Tanaka M, Ishiyama Y, Shimokubo T, Ichiki Y, Nakamura S, Kangawa K, Eto T. (1995) Plasma adrenomedullin in patients with primary aldosteronism. Am J Hypertens. 8:997-1000.

Khan AI, Kato J, Kitamura K, Kangawa K, Eto T. (1997a) Hypotensive effect of chronically infused adrenomedullin in conscious Wistar-Kyoto and spontaneously hypertensive rats. Clin Exp Pharmacol Physiol. 24:139-142.

Khan AI, Kato J, Ishiyama Y, Kitamura K, Kangawa K, Eto T. (1997b) Effect of chronically infused adrenomedullin in two-kidney, one-clip hypertensive rats. Eur J Pharmacol. 333:187-190.

Kitamura K, Kangawa K, Kawamoto M, Ichiki Y, Nakamura S, Matsuo H, and Eto

T. (1993a) Adrenomedullin: a novel hypotensive peptide isolated from human pheochromocytoma. Bioche Biophys Res Commun. 192:553-560.

Kitamura K, Sakata J, Kangawa K, Kojima M, Matsuo H, Eto T.(1993b) Cloning and characterization of cDNA encoding a precursor for human adrenomedullin. Biochem Biophys Res Commun. 194:720-725.

Kitamura K, Kangawa K, Kojima M, Ichiki Y, Matsuo H, Eto T. (1994) Complete amino acid sequence of porcine adrenomedullin and cloning of cDNA encoding its precursor. FEBS Lett. 338:306-310.

Kitamura K, Kato J, Kawamoto M, Tanaka M, Chino N, Kangawa K, Eto T. (1998) The intermediate form of glycine-extended adrenomedullin is the major circulating molecular form in human plasma. Biochem Biophys Res Commun. 244:551-555.

Kobayashi K, Kitamura K, Etoh T, Nagatomo Y, Takenaga M, Ishikawa T, Imamura T, Koiwaya Y, Eto T. (1996a) Increased plasma adrenomedullin levels in chronic congestive heart failure. Am Heart J. 131:994-998.

Kobayashi K, Kitamura K, Hirayama N, Date H, Kashiwagi T, Ikushima I, Hanada Y, Nagatomo Y, Takenaga M, Ishikawa T, Imamura T, Koiwaya Y, Eto T. (1996b) Increased plasma adrenomedullin in acute myocardial infarction. Am Heart J. 131:676-680.

Kohno M, Hanehira T, Kano H, Horio T, Yokokawa K, Ikeda M, Minami M, Yasunari K, Yoshikawa J. (1996) Plasma adrenomedullin concentrations in essential hypertension. Hypertension 27:102-107.

Lewis LK, Smith MW, Brennan SO, Yandle TG, Richards AM, Nicholls MG. (1997) Degradation of human adrenomedullin(1-52) by plasma membrane enzymes and identification of metabolites. Peptides. 18:733-739.

Lewis LK, Smith MW, Yandle TG, Richards AM, Nicholls MG. (1998) Adrenomedullin(1-52) measured in human plasma by radioimmunoassay: plasma concentration, adsorption, and storage. Clin Chem. 44:571-577.

Lisy O, Jougasaki M, Schirger JA, Chen HH, Barclay PT,Burnett JC Jr. (1998) Neutral endopeptidase inhibition potentiates the natriuretic actions of adrenomedullin. Am J Physiol. 275:F410-F414.

Meeran K, O'Shea D, Upton PD, Small CJ, Ghatei MA, Byfield PH, Bloom SR. (1997) Circulating adrenomedullin does not regulate systemic blood pressure but increases plasma prolactin after intravenous infusion in humans: a pharmacokinetic study. J Clin Endocrinol Metab. 82:95-100.

Minami J, Nishikimi T, Todoroki M, Kashiwakura C, Yagi H, Ono H, Horinaka S, Ishimitsu T, Kangawa K, Matsuoka H. (2002) Source of plasma adrenomedullin in patients with pheochromocytoma. Am J Hypertens. 15:994-997.

Miyao Y, Nishikimi T, Goto Y, Miyazaki S, Daikoku S, Morii I, Matsumoto T, Takishita S, Miyata A, Matsuo H, Kangawa K, Nonogi H. (1998) Increased plasma adrenomedullin levels in patients with acute myocardial infarction in proportion to the clinical severity. Heart. 79:39-44.

Mori Y, Nishikimi T, Kobayashi N, Ono H, Kangawa K, Matsuoka H. (2002) Long-term adrenomedullin infusion improves survival in malignant hypertensive rats. Hypertension. 40:107-113.

Morimoto A, Nishikimi T, Yoshihara F, Horio T, Nagaya N, Matsuo H, Dohi K, Kangawa K.(1999) Ventricular adrenomedullin levels correlate with the extent of cardiac hypertrophy in rats. Hypertension. 33:1146-1152.

Nagaya N, Nishikimi T, Uematsu M, Yoshitomi Y, Miyao Y, Miyazaki S, Goto Y, Kojima S, Kuramochi M, Matsuo H, Kangawa K, Nonogi H. (1999) Plasma adrenomedullin as an indicator of prognosis after acute myocardial infarction. Heart. 81:483-487.

Nagaya N, Nishikimi T, Uematsu M, Satoh T, Oya H, Kyotani S, Sakamaki F, Ueno K, Nakanishi N, Miyatake K, Kangawa K. (2000) Haemodynamic and hormonal effects of adrenomedullin in patients with pulmonary hypertension. Heart. 84:653-658.

Nagaya N, Goto Y, Satoh T, Sumida H, Kojima S, Miyatake K, Kangawa K. (2002) Intravenous adrenomedullin in myocardial function and energy metabolism in patients after myocardial infarction. J Cardiovasc Pharmacol. 39:754-760.

Nakamura R, Kato J, Kitamura K, Onitsuka H, Imamura T, Marutsuka K, Asada Y,

Kangawa K, Eto T. (2002) Beneficial effects of adrenomedullin on left ventricular remodeling after myocardial infarction in rats. Cardiovasc Res. 56:373-380.

Nishikimi T, Kitamura K, Saito Y, Shimada K, Ishimitsu T, Takamiya M, Kangawa K, Matsuo H, Eto T, Omae T, Matsuoka H. (1994) Clinical studies on the sites of production and clearance of circulating adrenomedullin in human subjects. Hypertension. 24:600-604.

Nishikimi T, Saito Y, Kitamura K, Ishimitsu T, Eto T, Kangawa K, Matsuo H, Omae T, Matsuoka H. (1995) Increased plasma levels of adrenomedullin in patients with heart failure. J Am Coll Cardiol. 26:1424-1431.

Nishikimi T, Matsuoka H, Ishikawa K, Yoshihara F, Kawano Y, Kitamura K, Saito Y, Kangawa K, Matsuo H, Omae T. (1996) Antihypertensive therapy reduces increased plasma levels of adrenomedullin and brain natriuretic peptide concomitant with regression of left ventricular hypertrophy in a patient with malignant hypertension. Hypertens Res. 19:97-101.

Nishikimi T, Nagata S, Sasaki T, Tomimoto S, Matsuoka H, Takishita S, Kitamura K, Miyata A, Matsuo H, Kangawa K. (1997) Plasma concentrations of adrenomedullin correlate with the extent of pulmonary hypertension in patients with mitral stenosis. Heart. 78:390-395.

Nishikimi T, Matsuoka H, Shimada K, Matsuo H, Kangawa K. (2000) Production and clearance sites of two molecular forms of adrenomedullin in human plasma. Am J Hypertens.13:1032-1034.

Nishikimi T, Horio T, Kohmoto Y, Yoshihara F, Nagaya N, Inenaga T, Saito M, Teranishi M, Nakamura M, Ohrui M, Kawano Y, Matsuo H, Ishimitsu T, Takishita S, Matsuoka H, Kangawa K. (2001a) Molecular forms of plasma and urinary adrenomedullin in normal, essential hypertension and chronic renal failure. J Hypertens 19:765-773.

Nishikimi T, Nagata S, Sasaki T, Yoshihara F, Nagaya N, Horio T, Matsuo H, Matsuoka H, Kangawa K. (2001b) The active molecular form of plasma adrenomedullin is extracted in the pulmonary circulation in patients with mitral stenosis: possible role of adrenomedullin in pulmonary hypertension.

Clin Sci. 100:61-66.

Nishikimi T, Mori Y, Kobayashi N, Tadokoro K, Wang X, Akimoto K, Yoshihara F, Kangawa K, Matsuoka H. (2002) Renoprotective effect of chronic adrenomedullin infusion in Dahl salt-sensitive rats. Hypertension. 39:1077-1082.

Nishikimi T, Tadokoro K, Mori Y, Wang X, Akimoto K, Yoshihara F, Minamino N, Kangawa K, Matsuoka H. (2003) Ventricular adrenomedullin system in the transition from LVH to heart failure in rats. Hypertension. 41:512-518.

Ohta H, Tsuji T, Asai S, Tanizaki S, Sasakura K, Teraoka H, Kitamura K, Kangawa K. (1999) A simple immunoradiometric assay for measuring the entire molecules of adrenomedullin in human plasma. Clin Chim Acta. 287:131-143.

Ohta H, Tsuji T, Asai S, Sasakura K, Teraoka H, Kitamura K, Kangawa K. (1999) One-step direct assay for mature-type adrenomedullin with monoclonal antibodies.ClinChem. 45:244-251.

Okumura H, Nagaya N, Itoh T, Okano I, Hino J, Mori K, Tsukamoto Y, Ishibashi-Ueda H, Miwa S, Tambara K, Toyokuni S, Yutani C, Kangawa K. (2004) Adrenomedullin infusion attenuates myocardial ischemia/reperfusion injury through the phosphatidylinositol 3-kinase/Akt-dependent pathway. Circulation. 109:242-248.

Pousset F, Masson F, Chavirovskaia O, Isnard R, Carayon A, Golmard JL, Lechat P, Thomas D, Komajda M. (2000) Plasma adrenomedullin, a new independent predictor of prognosis in patients with chronic heart failure. Eur Heart J. 21:1009-1014.

Richards AM, Nicholls MG, Yandle TG, Frampton C, Espiner EA, Turner JG, Buttimore RC, Lainchbury JG, Elliott JM, Ikram H, Crozier IG, Smyth DW. (1998) Plasma N-terminal pro-brain natriuretic peptide and adrenomedullin: new neurohormonal predictors of left ventricular function and prognosis after myocardial infarction. Circulation. 97:1921-1929.

Shimokubo T, Sakata J, Kitamura K, Kangawa K, Matsuo H, Eto T. (1996) Adrenomedullin: changes in circulating and cardiac tissue concentration in

Dahl salt-sensitive rats on a high-salt diet. Clin Exp Hypertens.18:949-961.

Sugo S, Minamino N, Shoji H, Kangawa K, Kitamura K, Eto T, Matsuo H. (1994) Production and secretion of adrenomedullin from vascular smooth muscle cells: augmented production by tumor necrosis factor-alpha. Biochem Biophys Res Commun. 203:719-726.

Sugo S, Minamino N, Kangawa K, Miyamoto K, Kitamura K, Sakata J, Eto T, Matsuo H. (1994) Endothelial cells actively synthesize and secrete adrenomedullin. Biochem Biophys Res Commun. 201:1160-1166.

Sumimoto T, Nishikimi T, Mukai M, Matsuzaki K, Murakami E, Takishita S, Miyata A, Matsuo H, Kangawa K. (1997) Plasma adrenomedullin concentrations and cardiac and arterial hypertrophy in hypertension. Hypertension. 30:741-745.

Szokodi I, Kinnunen P, Tavi P, Weckstrom M, Toth M, Ruskoaho H. (1998) Evidence for cAMP-independent mechanisms mediating the effects of adrenomedullin, a new inotropic peptide. Circulation. 97:1062- 1070.

Tadokoro K, Nishikimi T, Mori Y, Wang X, Akimoto K, Matsuoka H. (2003) Altered gene expression of adrenomedullin and its receptor system and molecular forms of tissue adrenomedullin in left ventricular hypertrophy induced by malignant hypertension. Regul Pept. 112:71-78.

Tsuruda T, Kato J, Kitamura K, Kuwasako K, Imamura T, Koiwaya Y, Tsuji T, Kangawa K, Eto T. (1998) Adrenomedullin: a possible autocrine or paracrine inhibitor of hypertrophy of cardiomyocytes. Hypertension. 31:505-510.

Tsuruda T, Kato J, Kitamura K, Kawamoto M, Kuwasako K, Imamura T, Koiwaya Y, Tsuji T, Kangawa K, Eto T.(1999) An autocrine or a paracrine role of adrenomedullin in modulating cardiac fibroblast growth. Cardiovasc Res. 43:958-967.

Yoshibayashi M, Kamiya T, Kitamura K, Saito Y, Kangawa K, Nishikimi T, Matsuoka H, Eto T, Matsuo H. (1997) Plasma levels of adrenomedullin in primary and secondary pulmonary hypertension in patients <20 years of age. Am J Cardiol. 79:1556-1558.

Yoshibayashi M, Kamiya T, Nishikimi T, Saito Y, Matsuo H, Kangawa K. (1999) Elevated plasma levels of adrenomedullin in congenital cyanotic heart disease. Clin Sci 96:543-547.

Yoshitomi Y, Nishikimi T, Kojima S, Kuramochi M, Takishita S, Matsuoka H, Miyata A, Matsuo H, Kangawa K. (1998) Plasma levels of adrenomedullin in patients with acute myocardial infarction. Clin Sci. 94:135-139.

Wang X, Nishikimi T, Akimoto K, Tadokoro K, Mori Y, Minamino N. (2003) Upregulation of ligand, receptor system, and amidating activity of adrenomedullin in left ventricular hypertrophy of severely hypertensive rats: effects of angiotensin-converting enzyme inhibitors and diuretic. J Hypertens. 21:1171-1181.

Watanabe K, Nishikimi T, Takamuro M, Yasuda K, Ishikawa Y, Tanabe S, Yamada O, Nagaya N, Matsuoka H, Kangawa K, Echigo S. (2003) Two molecular forms of adrenomedullin in congenital heart disease. Pediatr Cardiol. 24:559-565.

Yin H, Chao L, Chao J. (2004) Adrenomedullin protects against myocardial apoptosis after ischemia/reperfusion through activation of Akt-GSK signaling. Hypertension. 43:109-116.

7

ROLE OF ADRENOMEDULLIN IN CARDIOVASCULAR DISEASES

Johji Kato and Tanenao Eto

Miyazaki Medical College, University of Miyazaki, Miyazaki, Japan

INTRODUCTION

Adrenomedullin (AM) has a wide range of biological actions including vasodilatation, natriuresis, diuresis and inhibition of aldosterone secretion. Both the organs and tissues belonging to the cardiovascular system, such as the myocardium and vascular wall, were found to produce AM, and AM is present in the bloodstream in picomolar concentrations (Eto et al., 1999; Kitamura et al., 2002). Based upon its biological actions related to the homeostasis of cardiac and vascular functions (Table 1), AM is considered a humoral or locally acting factor modulating the development and progression of various cardiovascular diseases. Ever since the discovery of AM, efforts have been made to clarify the role of this bioactive peptide and a substantial amount of basic and clinical data has been accumulated. In this chapter, we comprehensively discuss the pathophysiological role of AM in cardiovascular diseases ranging from hypertension to sepsis, and examine the potential of AM as a therapeutic or diagnostic tool.

1. HYPERTENSION

(1) Plasma AM in essential hypertension

The biological action originally ascribed to AM was a blood pressure-lowering effect largely due to potent vasodilatation (Table 1) (Eto et al., 1999; Kitamura et al., 2002), therefore initial interest focused on the role of this bioactive peptide in the regulation of blood pressure.

Table 1. Biological actions of AM related to cardiovascular function

Organs or tissues	Biological actions
Heart	Inhibition of hypertrophy and fibrosis
Vasculature	Vasodilatation
	Stimulation of nitric oxide (NO) production
	Pulmonary Inhibition of endothelin production
Kidneys	Natriuresis, Diuresis
Lungs	Vasodilatation
Adrenal cortex	Inhibition of aldosterone secretion

Measurements with specific radioimmunoassays revealed plasma levels of AM to be higher in patients with essential hypertension than in normotensive controls (Eto et al., 1999). Cross-sectional, observational studies showed that the increase was related to blood pressure levels and to the severity of damage to target organs (Eto et al., 1999), suggesting a role for AM in lowering blood pressure. Unexpectedly, Kohno et al. (1996) demonstrated that plasma AM levels in untreated hypertensive patients remained unchanged after treatment with calcium channel blockers, despite a reduction in blood pressure. Instead, they found an intimate relationship between the plasma AM and serum creatinine levels, which suggests an increase in the plasma AM concentration is associated with impaired renal function (Kohno et al., 1996). Additionally, a single administration of angiotensin converting enzyme (ACE) inhibitor lowered blood pressure in a short period of time, but the plasma AM level remained unchanged (Kita et al., 1998). Thus, the increased plasma AM levels in patients with essential hypertension seem to be correlated not directly with blood pressure levels but with organ damage associated with an elevation of blood pressure. This, however, is not the case in patients with a more severe form of hypertension: plasma AM levels in patients with malignant hypertension rose to a much higher level, and dropped, along with blood pressure levels, following antihypertensive treatment within one to three weeks (Kato et al., 1999).

Immunoreactive AM in human plasma consists of two molecular forms: a mature form with an amidated C-terminal (mAM) and an intermediate form with an unamidated glycine-extended C-terminal (iAM) (Kitamura et al., 1998). In the process producing mAM, iAM is cleaved from the AM precursor peptide, and then converted to mAM by amidation enzymes. Plasma levels of mAM and iAM in hypertensive patients were similarly elevated, without a notable difference in the ratio of mAM to total AM (tAM), which is the sum of mAM and iAM, when compared with control subjects (Nishikimi et al., 2001). iAM itself is thought to have no biological effects, while a recent *ex vivo* study showed that iAM dilated rat aorta following its conversion to mAM probably in the aortic wall (Cao et al., 2003). The pathophysiological role of iAM in hypertension should be clarified further with experiments *in vivo*.

(2) Plasma AM in patients with pheochromocytoma and other forms of secondary hypertension

In addition to essential hypertension, there has been a number of reports on plasma AM levels in patients with secondary hypertension. Interest was aroused in plasma AM levels of patients with pheochromocytoma, which AM was originally isolated from and abundant AM expression is detected in (Kitamura et al., 1993). But unexpectedly, plasma AM levels were not necessarily higher in patients with pheochromocytoma than those with essential hypertension (Nishikimi et al., 1994). Moreover, no elevation of plasma AM was observed during the paroxysms of this disease despite the elevation of blood pressure and plasma catecholamines (Nishikimi et al., 1994). Comparable with this, there was no step-up in plasma AM concentrations of the adrenal vein compared with the inferior vena cava in primary aldosteronism (Kato et al., 1995). It is therefore unlikely that either pheochromocytoma or the adrenal medulla actively secretes AM into the blood stream, despite the abundance of AM peptide in these tissues. The organs or tissues contributing to plasma AM are discussed in more detail under AM production and its regulation of the heart failure section. Plasma AM levels are higher in patients with primary aldosteronism, renovascular hypertension and Cushing's syndrome than controls, as they are in those with essential hypertension (Kato et al., 1995; Kita et al., 1998; Letizia et al., 2000). A significant positive correlation was found between the plasma AM level and mean blood pressure in patients with primary aldosteronism (Kato et al., 1995). Meanwhile, no significant reduction in the plasma AM level was observed following surgical resection of an aldosterone-producing adrenal adenoma despite reduced blood pressure (Kita et al., 1998), a finding comparable with the effect of anti-hypertensive treatment on plasma AM levels in essential hypertensive patients (Kohno et al., 1996).

(3) Possible role of AM in hypertension

The intravenous injection of a bolus of AM lowers blood pressure largely through peripheral vasodilatation in anesthetized normotensive Wistar-Kyoto (WKY) rats and spontaneously hypertensive rats (SHR) (Ishiyama et al., 1995). The plasma AM concentration was shown to rise to a level 100-fold higher than the physiological concentration following such an injection (Ishiyama et al., 1995). Meanwhile, Khan et al. (1997a; 1997b) found that a relatively low dose of human AM infused continuously over two weeks exerted a prolonged lowering effect on blood pressure in SHR and in a rat model of renovascular hypertension at an AM level within the physiological range, suggesting a role for endogenous AM in reducing blood pressure. Further evidence supporting the anti-hypertensive role of endogenous AM is the elevation of blood pressure in heterozygotes of AM gene-knockout mice (Shindo et al., 2001). There have been a number of reports on the interaction between AM and the renin-angiotensin-aldosterone system. AM was found to reduce the secretion of aldosterone from the adrenal cortex both *in vitro* and *in vivo* (Kitamura et al., 2002). When infused over a relatively short period of time, AM raises plasma renin activity possibly via activation of the sympathetic nerve system, secondary to a reduction of blood pressure (Eto et al., 1999). Khan et al. (1997b) found, however, that not only the plasma aldosterone concentration but also the plasma renin activity in renovascular

hypertensive rats was reduced by prolonged AM infusion for two weeks.
As mentioned above, the increased plasma AM concentration appears largely related to damage to the target organ such as left ventricular hypertrophy, impaired renal function and arteriosclerosis. To investigate whether or not AM protects the target organs against hypertensive damages, two experimental approaches have so far been taken: chronic administration of AM and adenovirus-mediated overexpression of the AM gene. Using the former method, Nishikimi and his colleagues showed that AM lessened renal damage, reducing proteinuria, in a rat model of malignant hypertension, and attenuated the transition from left ventricular hypertrophy to heart failure in Dahl salt-sensitive hypertensive rats fed a high-salt diet (Nishikimi et al., 2003). Chao and coworkers demonstrated, by the latter approach, that the AM gene ameliorated renal damage, cardiac hypertrophy or fibrosis in rats with deoxycorticosterone acetate (DOCA) salt-induced and renovascular hypertension and in Dahl salt-sensitive hypertensive rats fed a high-salt diet (Chao et al., 2001). These findings suggest, taken together with the results of plasma AM measurements, that in hypertensive patients, AM functions to counteract the elevation in blood pressure and progression of organ damage associated with hypertension.

2. HEART FAILURE

(1) Plasma AM levels in heart failure

To examine the pathophysiological role of AM in heart failure, efforts have been made to measure plasma levels of this bioactive peptide. Consistent findings among these reports are as follows: plasma AM levels were higher in patients with chronic heart failure than in controls, and when patients were classified by the New York Heart Association (NYHA) functional class, the more severe the heart failure, the higher the plasma AM level (Eto et al., 1999). Interestingly, in comparison with other humoral factors or hemodynamic parameters, the plasma AM level was significantly correlated with pulmonary capillary wedge pressure, pulmonary artery pressure, plasma renin activity (PRA) and plasma levels of atrial and brain natriuretic peptides (ANP and BNP) (Kato et al., 1996; Kobayashi et al., 1996a). Moreover, according to Etoh et al. (1999), the elevated plasma levels gradually decreased following successful treatment, together with the levels of ANP and BNP, in patients with heart failure. These observational studies suggest an important role for AM in the pathophysiology of heart failure. Kobayashi et al. (1996a) subgrouped forty-nine patients with chronic heart failure based on the primary cause of heart disease, but failed to find any particular heart disease in which plasma AM rises higher than in the others. Therefore, the increased levels appear to be closely related to the degree of depressed cardiac function, not to the primary cause of heart failure. According to Hirayama et al. (1999b) who specifically measured mAM concentrations, plasma levels of mAM and iAM in heart failure patients were similarly elevated, without a notable difference in the ratio of mAM to total AM. In addition, plasma levels of the two molecular forms were found to similarly decrease following the treatment (Hirayama et al., 1999b). Pousset et al. (2000) measured plasma levels of AM in patients with chronic heart failure, and reported on long-term outcomes. They found that the higher the plasma level, the poorer the prognosis. Similar results were obtained by Richards et al. (2001), who carried out a follow-up study of patients with heart failure secondary to ischemic heart disease. In addition, treatment with β-adrenergic blockers was found to be more effective in patients with higher plasma levels of AM than in those with lower levels (Richards et al., 2001). It is therefore likely that the plasma AM level is not only a prognosticator in cases of heart failure but also a possible guide to selecting patients more likely to respond to treatment with β-blockers.

(2) AM production and its regulation

Both the AM peptide and gene expression have been detected in various organs and tissues, including the heart and blood vessels (Eto et al., 1999; Kitamura et al., 2002). Hirayama et al. (1999a) examined the plasma levels of AM in various sites of blood vessels in patients with ischemic heart disease. They found a step-up in the plasma AM level between the femoral artery and vein and between the aortic root and coronary sinus (Hirayama et al., 1999a). It has been reported that cultured cardiac cells and vascular smooth muscle or endothelial cells actively secrete the AM peptide into the culture medium (Kitamura et al., 2002; Uemura et al., 2002). Based also on these *in vitro* findings, both the heart and vasculature are assumed to partly supply the AM circulating in the blood of heart failure patients. On the other hand, there was found to be a step-down between the plasma AM levels of pulmonary artery and pulmonary capillary (Hirayama et al., 1999a). Despite having substantial levels of AM peptide and gene expression (Kitamura et al., 2002), the lung seems to be a target organ or a site for the clearance of circulating AM peptide rather than an AM-secreting organ. Consistent with this notion are reports of abundant expression of AM receptors in the lungs (Owji et al., 1995).

The mechanisms behind the elevation in plasma AM levels in heart failure patients are not fully understood, but presumably either humoral or mechanical factors are involved. According to a number of cell culture or animal studies, AM production is stimulated by various hormones or cytokines, such as angiotensin II, endothelin, aldosterone, IL-1β and TNF-α, in the cardiac tissues and vascular wall (Kitamura et al., 2002; Uemura et al., 2002; Kato et al., 2003). Mechanical stress to cardiac tissues has also been shown to increase AM production. For example, Tsuruda et al. (2000) found increased AM production on mechanical stretch in cultured cardiac myocytes isolated from the ventricles of neonatal rats. Consistent with this, cardiac ventricular AM expression was increased in rat models of pressure or volume overload to the heart (Kato et al., 2003). Hence, it is likely that augmented humoral and mechanical factors are involved in elevation of plasma AM levels in heart failure patients.

(3) AM actions in heart failure

Rademaker et al. (1997) reported the effects of AM in an ovine model of heart failure induced by cardiac ventricular pacing at a rate of 225 beats/min. In their experiments, intravenous AM administration lowered blood pressure and peripheral vascular resistance, while increasing cardiac output and creatinine clearance in kidneys, resulting in an increase of urinary sodium excretion. In addition, plasma levels and urinary excretion of cAMP were elevated, while the plasma aldosterone concentration was reduced by the AM administration (Rademaker et al., 1997). Based upon these findings, Rademaker et al. suggested the potential of AM as a therapeutic tool for heart failure. Effects of AM on human heart failure were reported by Nagaya et al. (2000b), who infused synthetic AM intravenously to patients with congestive heart failure of New York Heart Association (NYHA) functional class III or IV at a rate of 0.05 μg/kg/min. Similar to the animal studies, the AM infusion lowered systemic blood pressure and pulmonary capillary wedge pressure (PCWP), increasing the heart rate (HR) and cardiac index (CI). The extent of the PCWP reduction and CI increase was significantly greater, while the systemic blood pressure reduction was smaller, in the patients than controls. The smaller reduction of systemic blood pressure is comparable with the report by Nakamura et al. (1997) showing that the forearm vasodilator response to AM in patients with chronic heart failure is weaker than that of controls. Also, AM was found to increase urinary volume and sodium excretion in heart failure patients despite a reduction of systemic blood pressure (Nagaya et al., 2000b).

When discussing the pathophysiological roles of AM in heart failure, one needs to take local AM actions in the myocardium into account as well as the systemic effects described above. Both the AM peptide and AM mRNA were detected at substantial levels in cardiac atria and ventricles (Kitamura et al., 2002). As mentioned above, either pressure or volume overload to the heart has been shown to stimulate AM production in cardiac ventricles in animal experiments. Consistent with this is the increased AM peptide level in the failing myocardium of humans (Jougasaki et al., 1996). The roles of AM as a locally acting hormone have been studied by using cultured cells isolated from the cardiac ventricles of neonatal rats (Kato et al., 2003). These *in vitro* experiments showed that AM functions as an autocrine or paracrine hormone to inhibit the proliferation and collagen production of cardiac fibroblasts and to inhibit the hypertrophy of cardiomyocytes. Collectively, evidence accumulated to date supports the notion that AM is a humoral factor acting systematically or locally against progression of heart failure through its wide range of biological actions including vasodilatation, natriuresis, diuresis and inhibition of the renin-angiotensin-aldosterone system. The beneficial effects of AM imply the possibility of the clinical application of this bioactive peptide in treating patients with chronic heart failure.

3. ACUTE MYOCARDIAL INFARCTION

Acute myocardial infarction (AMI) should be mentioned as a heart disease in which notable changes of cardiac and plasma AM levels were observed (Kobayashi et al., 1996b; Nagaya et al., 2000a). The plasma AM level was found to be elevated in patients with AMI, particularly in cases complicated by pulmonary congestion, and to return to the basal level within one to three weeks (Kobayashi et al., 1996b). The elevated plasma levels are correlated with pulmonary capillary wedge pressure, pulmonary arterial pressure, right atrial pressure and heart rate in the AMI patients (Kobayashi et al., 1996b). Thus, similar to the plasma AM levels in chronic heart failure, the increased concentrations in AMI may be partly related to depressed cardiac function. The follow-up study showed that in patients with AMI, as plasma AM levels increased, so too did mortalities (Nagaya et al., 1999). In addition to the plasma levels, it should be noted that both the peptide and mRNA expression of AM were markedly increased in infarct and non-infarct left ventricles in a rat model with AMI (Nagaya et al., 2000a). According to cell culture experiments, the increased expression may partially be secondary to hypoxia of myocardial tissues (Kato et al., 2003).

To see the actions of AM in AMI, Nakamura et al. (2004) examined the effects of intraperitoneal infusion of recombinant human AM, started immediately after MI induction and continued for one weeks in rats. After the observational period for 8 weeks, they found an alleviation of left ventricular remodeling and heart failure with reduced left ventricular end-diastolic pressure. Using a rat model of ischemia-reperfusion myocardial injury, Okumura et al. (2004) showed the AM-induced reduction of infarct size with a preserved left ventricular function. Chao and colleagues reported that adenovirus-mediated AM gene delivery prior to myocardial ischemia-reperfusion injury attenuated the apoptosis of cardiac myocytes via an Akt-glycogen synthase kinase-dependent pathway (Yin et al., 2004). Anti-apoptotic effects, presumably cAMP-mediated, were also observed in cultured cardiac myocytes exposed to doxorubicin (Tokudome et al., 2002). These findings suggest a protective role of AM against myocardial ischemia, warranting further therapeutic, interventional studies for AMI not only in animal models but also in the clinical setting.

4. PULMONARY HYPERTENSION

As mentioned earlier, the AM peptide and mRNA are expressed in the lungs, where AM receptors are also detected (Owji et al., 1995; Kitamura et al., 2002). AM has been shown to dilate the pulmonary artery, thereby reducing pulmonary arterial pressure. To investigate the role of AM in pulmonary hypertension, Shimokubo et al. (1995) measured the plasma levels of AM in rats with monocrotaline-induced pulmonary hypertension. The plasma AM levels in this model were found to be higher than those in control rats. Nakanishi et al. (2004) found that AM mRNA and peptide were upregulated in the right ventricle and lungs of rats with pulmonary hypertension induced by hypobaric hypoxia. In addition to the upregulation, gene expression of the AM receptor components was found to be augmented in hypoxic rat lung (Qing et al., 2001). Kakishita et al. (1999) reported the plasma AM levels in patients with primary pulmonary hypertension or pulmonary hypertension secondary to chronic thromboembolism. In accord with the animal study, the AM levels in these patients were elevated compared to those of controls, and the increase was related to an elevation of mean pulmonary arterial pressure, right atrial pressure and pulmonary arterial resistance. These findings suggested AM acts against the elevation of pulmonary arterial pressure.

Yoshihara et al. (1998) reported the effects of continuous, subcutaneous administration of AM for three weeks in monocrotaline-induced pulmonary hypertension in rats. In their intervention experiments, AM partially inhibited an elevation of right ventricular pressure, alleviating right ventricular hypertrophy and the remodeling of pulmonary arterioles. This effect on the pulmonary vasculature is comparable with reports that AM inhibits the proliferation of cultured vascular smooth muscle cells isolated from rats or of those from human pulmonary artery (Kano et al., 1996; Upton et al 2001). Thus, AM seems to be a new therapeutic tool for treating patients with pulmonary hypertension; however, when infused intravenously, AM lowers not only pulmonary arterial pressure but also systemic blood pressure. In an attempt to avoid the effect on the systemic circulation, Nagaya et al. (2003) administered AM as an aerosol using an ultrasonic nebulizer in experimental pulmonary hypertension. Repeated inhalation effectively reduced pulmonary artery pressure and total pulmonary resistance, without affecting the systemic arterial pressure or heart rate. This novel approach seems promising for utilizing AM in the treatment of primary pulmonary hypertension, for which few effective medical treatments are currently available.

5. ARTERIOSCLEROSIS

Active AM secretion with AM mRNA expression was observed in cultured vascular endothelial and smooth muscle cells of rats and humans (Kitamura et al., 2002; Uemura et al., 2002), and as mentioned in the heart failure section, there is a body of evidence supporting production of AM in the human vasculature, which must partly contribute to the plasma AM level (Hirayama et al., 1999a). Kuwasako et al. (1997) found a possible association between plasma AM levels and endothelial damage by comparing the plasma levels of AM with those of endothelin and thrombomodulin, markers of endothelial damage, in patients with cerebrovascular disease. Similarly, in patients with chronic ischemic stroke, the increased plasma AM level was shown to be associated with the degree of carotid atherosclerosis (Shinomiya et al., 2001). Recently, Suzuki et al. (2004) reported that the plasma AM concentration was elevated in

patients with peripheral arterial occlusive disease in proportion to its severity. These findings are indirect, but indicative of a possible pathophysiological role of AM in arteriosclerotic vascular disease.
To clarify the role of AM in arteriosclerosis, its effects on the proliferation and migration of cultured vascular smooth muscle cells (VSMC) have been examined, but the results seem conflicting. AM was found to inhibit the agonist-induced proliferation and migration of cultured VSMC (Horio et al., 1995; Kano et al., 1996), but conversely, Iwasaki et al. (1998) reported that AM stimulated VSMC proliferation by activating a MAP kinase cascade. On the other hand, there is a significant amount of evidence suggesting a protective role for AM in the vascular endothelium. Shichiri et al. (1999) found an inhibitory effect of AM on apoptosis of cultured endothelial cells, an action possibly mediated by induction of max protein. Recently, Hippenstiel et al. (2002) reported that AM suppressed the agonist-induced permeability of human vascular endothelial cells. In line with these findings, inhibitory actions of AM on the development of atherosclerotic vascular lesions were reported in animal models or in transgenic mice overexpressing the AM gene (AM-Tg mice). For example, periarterial cuff-induced neointimal formation was inhibited by a periarterial, adenovirus-mediated delivery of the AM gene (Yamasaki et al., 2003), and it was also less extensive in AM-Tg mice compared with wild type mice (Imai et al., 2002). Moreover, the aorta of apoE-knockout mice overexpressing the AM gene showed significantly less fatty streak formation than those without AM overexpression (Imai et al., 2002). Thus, clinical and experimental findings suggest that AM protects against the progression of arteriosclerosis, but this important issue needs to be clarified further.

6. RENAL DISEASES

(1) AM production and its actions in kidneys

Several lines of evidence suggest a role for AM in the regulation of renal function. When infused into experimental animals, AM has been shown to increase urinary volume and sodium excretion, increasing renal blood flow, with no or a slight change in the glomerular filtration rate (Eto et al., 2001). Ebara et al. (1994) reported the natriuretic action of AM resulting from inhibition of tubular sodium reabsorption in rats presumably at a plasma AM level within the physiological range. In addition to the possible action of circulating AM on the kidneys, the AM peptide and mRNA are present in renal tubular cells, mesangial cells and vascular endothelial and smooth muscle cells of animals and humans (Eto et al., 1999; Eto et al., 2001), and expression of the AM receptors is also shown (Nagae et al., 2000). These *in vitro* data suggest an autocrine or paracrine role for AM in the modulation of renal tubular or glomerular function.

(2) Plasma AM in chronic glomerulonephritis (CGN)

Kubo et al. (1998) reported that plasma AM levels in patients with IgA nephropathy were increased in correlation with serum creatinine levels. Conversely, urinary AM levels were lower in the patients than controls, and interestingly, a negative correlation was noted between the urinary AM level and biopsy evidence of disease activity (Kubo et al., 1998). By separately analyzing mAM and iAM in plasma of CGN patients, the mAM level in the patients was found to be higher than in controls, without a significant difference in the iAM levels (Kinoshita et al., 2000). Meanwhile, in this series of patients, a significant reduction was noted in urinary iAM excretion but not in urinary mAM. It is possible that nephrons contributc to urinary AM because of the AM production in glomeruli and tubules (Eto et al., 2001). Although cell culture experiments suggest a protective role for AM in glomeruli (Chini et al., 1997), there is currently little *in vivo* data available to discuss the role of AM in CGN.

(3) Plasma AM in chronic renal failure and end-stage renal disease

Irrespective of the basal renal disease, the plasma AM concentration progressively increased in proportion to the impairment of renal function in patients with chronic renal failure (CRF) (Eto et al., 2001).

Both mAM and iAM levels are elevated in CRF patients without a significant alteration in the ratio of mAM to total AM (Ishihara et al., 1999). Since peptide hormones and small fragments of peptides are metabolized in the kidneys, the possibility of a decreased clearance of AM should be taken into account as an explanation for the increased AM concentration. Meanwhile, according to the report by Nishikimi et al. (1994), no significant step-down of the plasma AM levels was noted between the renal artery and vein of hypertensive patients. This finding does not support the notion that the kidneys are the major clearance sites of AM circulating in the blood. The elevated plasma AM levels in patients with CRF may not be simply attributed to the impaired renal function.

To understand the role of AM, it is essential to discuss whether or not its effects are altered in patients with CRF when compared with those with normal renal function. McGregor et al. (2001) examined the effects of AM infused intravenously over four hours in patients with CRF secondary to IgA nephropathy. Interestingly, despite the increased plasma levels of endogenous AM and reduced renal function, both hypotensive and renal responses to AM in the CRF patients were not necessarily attenuated compared with those of healthy volunteers or uncomplicated essential hypertensive patients. It was reported that in a rat model of obstructive nephropathy, gene expression of the AM receptor proteins was markedly upregulated in the obstructed kidney (Nagae et al., 2000). Alteration of the AM effecter system may also occur in patients with CRF. These findings suggest the possible participation of AM in the mechanisms counteracting the elevation of blood pressure and fluid volume retention in patients with CRF.

There are a number of reports on the plasma AM level in patients with end-stage renal disease (ESRD) and on its change with hemodialysis (HD). A consistent finding among these reports is that plasma AM levels are markedly increased in ESRD patients, but there is some inconsistency regarding changes in plasma levels following HD. Some investigators found reduced plasma AM concentrations in an HD session (Mallamaci et al., 1998), while others reported that AM levels remained unchanged (Washimine et al., 1995). The plasma AM levels were shown to be reduced by HD with a high-flux dialyzer, but not with a low-flux dialyzer (Yamasaki et al., 2001). Kanozawa et al. (2002) reported that AM levels were lowered in patients undergoing ultrafiltration (UF), but remained unchanged in those without UF. The discrepancy in changes of plasma AM levels in the HD patients may be partly explained by differences in subtracted fluid volume or in the types of dialyzer used. In any case, the increased plasma levels suggest a possible modulation of blood pressure and fluid volume by AM in HD patients.

7. SEPSIS

Since the discovery of AM, vigorous efforts have been made to examine the pathophysiological role of this bioactive peptide by measuring its plasma levels in various diseases, among which a marked elevation was observed in plasma of patients with sepsis (Nishio et al., 1997). Consistent results were obtained in rat models of sepsis induced by lipopolysaccharide (LPS) injection and by ligation and puncture of the cecum (Matsui et al., 2001; Zhou et al., 2002). In these animal models, both the AM mRNA expression and peptide levels were markedly upregulated in a wide range of organs and tissues, such as heart, lungs, aorta and small intestine, which are thought to contribute to the elevated plasma AM concentrations (Matsui et al., 2001; Zhou et al., 2001). It was documented that AM production and secretion by cultured vascular cells was increased not only by LPS but also by interleukin-1β (IL-1β) and tumor necrosis factor-α (TNF-α), cytokines that have an important role in sepsis (Kitamura et al., 2002). The augmented AM secretion by these cytokines was also observed in cardiac fibroblasts and a macrophage-derived cell line (Kubo et al., 1998; Kato et al., 2003). These findings are comparable with the report by Ueda et al. (1999), where a significant correlation was found between plasma AM and TNF-α levels in patients with septic shock. The plasma AM level in septic patients was found to decline during the recovery and to be correlated positively with the multiple organ damage score and with the prognosis of the patients (Ueda et al., 1999). In addition, an intimate relationship was observed between the elevation in the plasma AM levels and reduction in the peripheral vascular resistance that occasionally results in refractory hypotension (Nishio et al., 1997). These findings suggest that the plasma AM level can be a useful marker in evaluating the severity of sepsis.

Because of the potent vasodilator action of AM, the increased plasma level in septic patients was considered to be involved in the refractory hypotension. Indeed, Hyvelin et al. (2002) reported an improved survival of rats with LPS-induced sepsis following a blockade of AM's action by anti-AM antiserum. Meanwhile, this was not always the case in other reports. According to Shindo et al. (2000), transgenic mice overexpressing AM turned out to be more sepsis-resistant than their wild-type littermates, showing a smaller BP reduction, higher survival and less organ damage following LPS injection. Wang and his colleagues found a reduced vasodilator response to AM in aorta from septic rats, where AM binding protein-1 (AMBP-1), a protein identified as complement factor H, was down-regulated, and interestingly, this hyporesponsiveness was restored by supplying AMBP-1 (Zhou et al., 2002). Moreover, the same group showed that intravenous administration of AM with AMBP-1 into a rat model of sepsis prevented the transition from the hyperdynamic to the hypodynamic phase, stabilizing hemodynamic parameters and reducing plasma levels of TNF-α, IL-1β and LI-6, and finally improved the mortality (Yang et al., 2002). Though the precise mechanism of AMBP-1 actions remains to be clarified, these findings suggest that AM functions, with or without AMBP-1, as a protective factor at least in the relatively early phase of sepsis.

PERSPECTIVES

Ten years has passed since AM was discovered as a novel vasodilator peptide. During this decade, much research, basic and clinical, has been done to clarify its role in the homeostasis of cardiovascular functions, and a substantial amount of data has been accumulated in this field. Research on AM now seems to be entering a new phase, with clinical benefits to be examined and specified. For instance, the beneficial effects of AM are about to be tested in patients with acute myocardial infarction and in those with pulmonary hypertension. It appears certain that further data will be provided as to the clinical application of AM in diagnosing or treating patients with cardiovascular diseases.

REFERENCES

Cao YN, Kitamura K, Ito K, Kato J, Hashida S, Morishita K, and Eto T. (2003) Glycine-extended adrenomedullin exerts vasodilator effect through amidation in the rat aorta. Regul Pept 113:109-114.

Chao J, Kato K, Zhang JJ, Dobrzynski E, Wang C, Agata J, Chao L. (2001) Human adrenomedullin gene delivery protects against cardiovascular remodeling and renal injury. Peptides 22:1731-1737.

Chini EN, Chini CCS, Bolliger C, Jougasaki M, Grande JP, Burnett JC Jr, and Dousa TP. (1997) Cytoprotective effects of adrenomedullin in glomerular cell injury: central role of cAMP signaling pathway. Kidney Int 52:917-925.

Ebara T, Miura K, Okumura M, Matsuura T, Kim S, Yukimura T, and Iwao H. (1994) Effect of adrenomedullin on renal hemodynamics and functions in dogs. Eur J Pharmacol 263:69-73.

Eto T, Kitamura K, and Kato J. (1999) Biological and clinical roles of adrenomedullin in circulation control and cardiovascular diseases. Clin Exp Pharmacol Physiol 26:371-380.

Eto T and Kitamura K. (2001) Adrenomedullin and its role in renal diseases. Nephron 89:121-134.

Etoh T, Kato J, Takenaga M, Imamura T, Kitamura K, Koiwaya Y, and Eto T. (1999) Differential hormonal profiles of adrenomedullin and proadrenomedullin N-terminal 20 peptide in patients with heart failure and effect of treatment on their plasma levels. Clin Cardiol 22:113-117.

Hippenstiel S, Witzenrath M, Schmeck B, Hocke A, Krisp M, Krull M, Seybold J, Seeger W, Rascher W, Schutte H, and Suttorp N. (2002) Adrenomedullin reduces endothelial hyperpermeability. Circ Res 91: 618-625.

Hirayama N, Kitamura K, Imamura T, Kato J, Koiwaya Y, and Eto T. (1999a) Secretion and clearance of the mature form of adrenomedullin in humans. Life Sci 64:2505-2509.

Hirayama N, Kitamura K, Imamura T, Kato J, Koiwaya Y, Tsuji T, Kangawa K, and Eto T. (1999b) Molecular forms of circulating adrenomedullin in patients with congestive heart failure. J

Endocrinol 160:297-303.
Horio T, Kohno M, Kano H, Ikeda M, Yasunari K, Yokokawa K, Minami M, and Takeda T. (1995) Adrenomedullin as a novel antimigration factor of vascular smooth muscle cells. Circ Res 77:660-664.
Hyvelin JM, Shan Q, and Bourreau JP. (2002) Adrenomedullin: a cardiac depressant factor in septic shock. J Card Surg 17: 328-335.
Imai Y, Shindo T, Maemura K, Sata M, Saito Y, Kurihara Y, Akishita M, Osuga J, Ishibashi S, Tobe K, Morita H, Oh-hashi Y, Suzuki T, Maekawa H, Kangawa K, Minamino N, Yazaki Y, Nagai R, and Kurihara H. (2002) Resistance to neointimal hyperplasia and fatty streak formation in mice with adrenomedullin overexpression. Arterioscler Thromb Vasc Biol 22:1310-1315.
Ishihara T, Yokota N, Hisanaga S, Fujimoto S, Hirayama N, Kato J, Kitamura K, and Eto T. (1999) Increased plasma levels of mature form of adrenomedullin in patients with chronic renal failure. Clin Nephrol 52:119-123.
Ishiyama Y, Kitamura K, Ichiki Y, Sakata J, Kida O, Kangawa K, and Eto T. (1995) Haemodynamic responses to rat adrenomedullin in anaesthetized spontaneously hypertensive rats. Clin Exp Pharmacol Physiol 22:614-618.
Iwasaki H, Eguchi S, Shichiri M, Marumo F, and Hirata Y. (1998) Adrenomedullin as a novel growth-promoting factor for cultured vascular smooth muscle cells: role of tyrosine kinase-mediated mitogen-activated protein kinase activation. Endocrinology 139:3432-3441.
Jougasaki M, Rodeheffer RJ, Redfield MM, Yamamoto K, Wei CM, McKinley LJ, and Burnett JC Jr. (1996) Cardiac secretion of adrenomedullin in human heart failure. J Clin Invest 97:2370-2376.
Kakishita M, Nishikimi T, Okano Y, Satoh T, Kyotani S, Nagaya N, Fukushima K, Nakanishi N, Takishita S, Miyata A, Kangawa K, Matsuo H, and Kunieda T. (1999) Increased plasma levels of adrenomedullin in patients with pulmonary hypertension. Clin Sci 96:33-39.
Kano H, Kohno M, Yasunari K, Yokokawa K, Horio T, Ikeda M, Minami M, Hanehira T, Takeda T, and Yoshikawa J. (1996) Adrenomedullin as a novel antiproliferative factor of vascular smooth muscle cells. J Hypertens 14:209-213.
Kanozawa K, Shimosawa T, Nagasawa R, Matsuda A, Kato H, Matsumura O, Mitarai T, Isoda K, and Fujita T. (2002) Mature form of adrenomedullin is a useful marker to evaluate blood volume in hemodialysis patients. Am J Kidney Dis 40:794-801.
Kato J, Kitamura K, Kuwasako K, Tanaka M, Ishiyama Y, Shimokubo T,

Ichiki Y, Nakamura S, Kangawa K, and Eto T. (1995) Plasma adrenomedullin in patients with primary aldosteronism. Am J Hypertens 8:997-1000.

Kato J, Kobayashi K, Etoh T, Tanaka M, Kitamura K, Imamura T, Koiwaya Y, Kangawa K, and Eto T. (1996) Plasma adrenomedullin concentration in patients with heart failure. J Clin Endocrinol Metab 81:180-183.

Kato J, Kitamura K, Matsui E, Tanaka M, Ishizaka Y, Kita T, Kangawa K, and Eto T. (1999) Plasma adrenomedullin and natriuretic peptides in patients with essential or malignant hypertension. Hypertens Res 22:61-65.

Kato J, Tsuruda T, Kitamura K, and Eto T. (2003) Adrenomedullin: a possible autocrine or paracrine hormone in the cardiac ventricles. Hypertens Res 26:S113-S119.

Khan AI, Kato J, Kitamura K, Kangawa K, and Eto T. (1997a) Hypotensive effect of chronically infused adrenomedullin in conscious Wistar-Kyoto and spontaneously hypertensive rats. Clin Exp Pharmacol Physiol 24:139-142.

Khan AI, Kato J, Ishiyama Y, Kitamura K, Kangawa K, and Eto T. (1997b) Effect of chronically infused adrenomedullin in two-kidney, one-clip hypertensive rats. Eur J Pharmacol 333:187-190.

Kinoshita H, Fujimoto S, Kitamura K, Matsuura Y, Uezono S, Hisanaga S, and Eto T. (2000) Increased plasma levels of mature adrenomedullin in chronic glomerulonephritis. Nephron 86:333-338.

Kita T, Kitamura K, Kuwasako K, Kawamoto M, and Eto T. (1998) Short-term modulation of the renin-angiotensin system does not alter plasma adrenomedullin concentration in humans. J Hypertens 16:2057-2062.

Kitamura K, Kangawa K, Kawamoto M, Ichiki Y, Nakamura S, Matsuo H, and Eto T. (1993) Adrenomedullin: a novel hypotensive peptide isolated from human pheochromocytoma. Biochem Biophys Res Commun 192:553-560.

Kitamura K, Kato J, Kawamoto M, Tanaka M, Chino N, Kangawa K, and Eto T. (1998) The intermediate form of glycine-extended adrenomedullin is the major circulating molecular form in human plasma. Biochem Biophys Res Commun 244:551-555.

Kitamura K, Kangawa K, and Eto T. (2002) Adrenomedullin and PAMP: discovery, structures, and cardiovascular functions. Microsc Res Tech 57:3-13.

Kobayashi K, Kitamura K, Etoh T, Nagatomo Y, Takenaga M, Ishikawa T, Imamura T, Koiwaya Y, and Eto T. (1996a) Increased plasma adrenomedullin levels in chronic congestive heart failure. Am Heart J 131:994-998.

Kobayashi K, Kitamura K, Hirayama N, Date H, Kashiwagi T, Ikushima I, Hanada Y, Nagatomo Y, Takenaga M, Ishikawa T, Imamura T, Koiwaya Y, and Eto T. (1996b) Increased plasma adrenomedullin in acute myocardial infarction. Am Heart J 131:676-680.

Kohno M, Hanehira T, Kano H, Horio T, Yokokawa K, Ikeda M, Minami M, Yasunari K, and Yoshikawa J. (1996) Plasma adrenomedullin concentrations in essential hypertension. Hypertension 27:102-107.

Kubo A, Iwano M, Minamino N, Sato H, Nishino T, Hirata E, Akai Y, Shiiki H, Kitamura K, Kangawa K, Matsuo H, and Dohi K. (1998) Measurement of plasma and urinary adrenomedullin in patients with IgA nephropathy. Nephron 78:389-394.

Kubo A, Minamino N, Isumi Y, Katafuchi T, Kangawa K, Dohi K, and Matsuo H. (1998) Production of adrenomedullin in macrophage cell line and peritoneal macrophage. J Biol Chem 273:16730-16738.

Kuwasako K, Kida O, Kitamura K, Kato J, and Eto T. (1997) Plasma adrenomedullin in cerebrovascular disease: a possible indicator of endothelial injury. Int Angiol 16:272-279.

Letizia C, Di Iorio R, De Toma G, Marinoni E, Cerci S, Celi M, Subioli S, and D'Erasmo E. (2000) Circulating adrenomedullin is increased in patients with corticotropin-dependent Cushing's syndrome due to pituitary adenoma. Metabolism 49:760-763.

Mallamaci F, Zoccali C, Parlongo S, Cutrupi S, Tripepi G, and Postorino M. (1998) Plasma adrenomedullin during acute changes in intravascular volume in hemodialysis patients. Kidney Int 54:1697-1703.

Matsui E, Kitamura K, Yoshida M, Kato J, Asada Y, Sumiyoshi A, and Eto T. (2001) Biosynthesis and secretion of adrenomedullin and proadrenomedullin N-terminal 20 peptide in a rat model of endotoxin shock. Hypertens Res 24:543-549.

McGregor DO, Troughton RW, Frampton C, Lynn KL, Yandle T, Richards AM, and Nicholls MG. (2001) Hypotensive and natriuretic actions of adrenomedullin in subjects with chronic renal impairment. Hypertension 37:1279-1284.

Nagae T, Mukoyama M, Sugawara A, Mori K, Yahata K, Kasahara M, Suganami T, Makino H, Fujinaga Y, Yoshioka T, Tanaka I, and Nakao K. (2000) Rat receptor-activity-modifying proteins (RAMPs) for adrenomedullin/CGRP receptor: cloning and upregulation in obstructive nephropathy. Biochem Biophys Res Commun 270:89-93.

Nagaya N, Nishikimi T, Uematsu M, Yoshitomi Y, Miyao Y, Miyazaki S, Goto Y, Kojima S, Kuramochi M, Matsuo H, Kangawa K, and Nonogi H. (1999) Plasma adrenomedullin as an indicator of

prognosis after acute myocardial infarction. Heart 81:483-487.
Nagaya N, Nishikimi T, Yoshihara F, Horio T, Morimoto A, and Kangawa K. (2000a) Cardiac adrenomedullin gene expression and peptide accumulation after acute myocardial infarction in rats. Am J Physiol Regul Integr Comp Physiol 278:R1019-R1026.
Nagaya N, Satoh T, Nishikimi T, Uematsu M, Furuichi S, Sakamaki F, Oya H, Kyotani S, Nakanishi N, Goto Y, Masuda Y, Miyatake K, and Kangawa K. (2000b) Hemodynamic, renal, and hormonal effects of adrenomedullin infusion in patients with congestive heart failure. Circulation 101:498-503.
Nagaya N, Okumura H, Uematsu M, Shimizu W, Ono F, Shirai M, Mori H, Miyatake K, and Kangawa K. (2003) Repeated inhalation of adrenomedullin ameliorates pulmonary hypertension and survival in monocrotaline rats. Am J Physiol Heart Circ Physiol 285: H2125-H2131.
Nakamura M, Yoshida H, Makita S, Arakawa N, Niinuma H, and Hiramori K. (1997) Potent and long-lasting vasodilatory effects of adrenomedullin in humans. Comparisons between normal subjects and patients with chronic heart failure. Circulation 95:1214-1221.
Nakamura R, Kato J, Kitamura K, Onitsuka H, Imamura T, Cao Y, Marutsuka K, Asada Y, Kangawa K, and Eto T. (2004) Adrenomedullin administration immediately after myocardial infarction ameliorates progression of heart failure in rats. Circulation 110:426-431.
Nakanishi K, Osada H, Uenoyama M, Kanazawa F, Ohrui N, Masaki Y, Hayashi T, Kanatani Y, Ikeda T, and Kawai T. (2004) Expressions of adrenomedullin mRNA and protein in rats with hypobaric hypoxia-induced pulmonary hypertension. Am J Physiol Heart Circ Physiol 286: H2159-H2168.
Nishikimi T, Kitamura K, Saito Y, Shimada K, Ishimitsu T, Takamiya M, Kangawa K, Matsuo H, Eto T, Omae T, and Matsuoka H. (1994) Clinical studies on the sites of production and clearance of circulating adrenomedullin in human subjects. Hypertension 24:600-604.
Nishikimi T, Horio T, Kohmoto Y, Yoshihara F, Nagaya N, Inenaga T, Saito M, Teranishi M, Nakamura M, Ohrui M, Kawano Y, Matsuo H, Ishimitsu T, Takishita S, Matsuoka H, and Kangawa K. (2001) Molecular forms of plasma and urinary adrenomedullin in normal, essential hypertension and chronic renal failure. J Hypertens 19:765-773.
Nishikimi T, Yoshihara F, Mori Y, Kangawa K, and Matsuoka H. (2003) Cardioprotective effect of adrenomedullin in heart failure. Hypertens Res 26:S121-S127.

Nishio K, Akai Y, Murao Y, Doi N, Ueda S, Tabuse H, Miyamoto S, Dohi K, Minamino N, Shoji H, Kitamura K, Kangawa K, and Matsuo H. (1997) Increased plasma concentrations of adrenomedullin correlate with relaxation of vascular tone in patients with septic shock. Crit Care Med 25: 953-957.

Okumura H, Nagaya N, Itoh T, Okano I, Hino J, Mori K, Tsukamoto Y, Ishibashi-Ueda H, Miwa S, Tambara K, Toyokuni S, Yutani C, and Kangawa K. (2004) Adrenomedullin infusion attenuates myocardial ischemia/reperfusion injury through the phosphatidylinositol 3-kinase/Akt-dependent pathway. Circulation 109:242-248.

Owji AA, Smith DM, Coppock HA, Morgan DGA, Bhogal R, Ghatei MA, and Bloom SR. (1995) An abundant and specific binding site for the novel vasodilator adrenomedullin in the rat. Endocrinology 136:2127-2134.

Qing X, Svaren J, and Keith IM. (2001) mRNA expression of novel CGRP1 receptors and their activity-modifying proteins in hypoxic rat lung. Am J Physiol Lung Cell Mol Physiol 280: L547-L554.

Pousset F, Masson F, Chavirovskaia O, Isnard R, Carayon A, Golmard JL, Lechat P, Thomas D, and Komajda M. (2000) Plasma adrenomedullin, a new independent predictor of prognosis in patients with chronic heart failure. Eur Heart J 21:1009-1014.

Rademaker MT, Charles CJ, Lewis LK, Yandle TG, Cooper GJS, Coy DH, Richards AM, and Nicholls MG. (1997) Beneficial hemodynamic and renal effects of adrenomedullin in an ovine model of heart failure. Circulation 96:1983-1990.

Richards AM, Doughty R, Nicholls MG, MacMahon S, Sharpe N, Murphy J, Espiner EA, Frampton C, and Yandle TG; Australia-New Zealand Heart Failure Group. (2001) Plasma N-terminal pro-brain natriuretic peptide and adrenomedullin: prognostic utility and prediction of benefit from carvedilol in chronic ischemic left ventricular dysfunction. J Am Coll Cardiol 37:1781-1787.

Shichiri M, Kato H, Doi M, Marumo F, and Hirata Y. (1999) Induction of max by adrenomedullin and calcitonin gene-related peptide antagonizes endothelial apoptosis. Mol Endocrinol 13:1353-1363.

Shimokubo T, Sakata J, Kitamura K, Kangawa K, Matsuo H, and Eto T. (1995) Augmented adrenomedullin concentrations in right ventricle and plasma of experimental pulmonary hypertension. Life Sci 57:1771-1779.

Shindo T, Kurihara H, Maemura K, Kurihara Y, Kuwaki T, Izumida T, Minamino N, Ju KH, Morita H, Oh-hashi Y, Kumada M, Kangawa K, Nagai R, and Yazaki Y. (2000) Hypotension and resistance to lipopolysaccharide-induced shock in transgenic mice overexpressing adrenomedullin in their vasculature. Circulation 101:2309-2316.

Shindo T, Kurihara Y, Nishimatsu H, Moriyama N, Kakoki M, Wang Y, Imai Y, Ebihara A, Kuwaki T, Ju KH, Minamino N, Kangawa K, Ishikawa T, Fukuda M, Akimoto Y, Kawakami H, Imai T, Morita H, Yazaki Y, Nagai R, Hirata Y, and Kurihara H. (2001) Vascular abnormalities and elevated blood pressure in mice lacking adrenomedullin gene. Circulation 104:1964-1971.

Shinomiya K, Ohmori K, Ohyama H, Hosomi N, Takahashi T, Osaka K, and Kohno M. (2001) Association of plasma adrenomedullin with carotid atherosclerosis in chronic ischemic stroke. Peptides 22:1873-1880.

Suzuki Y, Horio T, Hayashi T, Nonogi H, Kitamura K, Eto T, Kangawa K, and Kawano Y. (2004) Plasma adrenomedullin concentration is increased in patients with peripheral arterial occlusive disease associated with vascular inflammation. Regul Pept 118:99-104.

Tokudome T, Horio T, Yoshihara F, Suga S, Kawano Y, Kohno M, and Kangawa K. (2002) Adrenomedullin inhibits doxorubicin-induced cultured rat cardiac myocyte apoptosis via a cAMP-dependent mechanism. Endocrinology 143:3515-3521.

Tsuruda T, Kato J, Kitamura K, Imamura T, Koiwaya Y, Kangawa K, Komuro I, Yazaki Y, and Eto T. (2000) Enhanced adrenomedullin production by mechanical stretching in cultured rat cardiomyocytes. Hypertension 35:1210-1214.

Ueda S, Nishio K, Minamino N, Kubo A, Akai Y, Kangawa K, Matsuo H, Fujimura Y, Yoshioka A, Masui K, Doi N, Murao Y, and Miyamoto S. (1999) Increased plasma levels of adrenomedullin in patients with systemic inflammatory response syndrome. Am J Respir Crit Care Med 160:132-136.

Uemura T, Kato J, Kuwasako K, Kitamura K, Kangawa K, and Eto T. (2002) Aldosterone augments adrenomedullin production without stimulating pro-adrenomedullin N-terminal 20 peptide secretion in vascular smooth muscle cells. J Hypertens 20:1209-1214.

Upton PD, Wharton J, Coppock H, Davie N, Yang X, Yacoub MH, Ghatei MA, Polak JM, Bloom SR, Smith DM, and Morrell NW. (2001) Adrenomedullin expression and growth inhibitory effects in distinct pulmonary artery smooth muscle cell subpopulations. Am J Respir Cell Mol Biol 24: 170-178.

Washimine H, Yamamoto Y, Kitamura K, Tanaka M, Ichiki Y, Kangawa K, Matsuo H, and Eto T. (1995) Plasma concentration of human adrenomedullin in patients on hemodialysis. Clin Nephrol 44:389-393.

Yamasaki H, Nagake Y, Akagi S, Sugimoto T, Ichikawa H, and Makino H.

(2001) Plasma adrenomedullin levels in patients on hemodialysis. Nephron 89:20-25.

Yamasaki M, Kawai J, Nakaoka T, Ogita T, Tojo A, and Fujita T. (2003) Adrenomedullin overexpression to inhibit cuff-induced arterial intimal formation. Hypertension 41:302-307.

Yang S, Zhou M, Fowler DE, and Wang P. (2002) Mechanisms of the beneficial effect of adrenomedullin and adrenomedullin-binding protein-1 in sepsis: down-regulation of proinflammatory cytokines. Crit Care Med 30: 2729-2735.

Yin H, Chao L, and Chao J. (2004) Adrenomedullin protects against myocardial apoptosis after ischemia/reperfusion through activation of Akt-GSK signaling. Hypertension 43:109-116.

Yoshihara F, Nishikimi T, Horio T, Yutani C, Takishita S, Matsuo H, Ohe T, and Kangawa K. (1998) Chronic infusion of adrenomedullin reduces pulmonary hypertension and lessens right ventricular hypertrophy in rats administered monocrotaline. Eur J Pharmacol 355:33-39.

Zhou M, Chaudry IH, and Wang P. (2001) The small intestine is an important source of adrenomedullin release during polymicrobial sepsis. Am J Physiol Regul Integr Comp Physiol 281: R654-R660.

Zhou M, Ba ZF, Chaudry IH, and Wang P. (2002) Adrenomedullin binding protein-1 modulates vascular responsiveness to adrenomedullin in late sepsis. Am J Physiol Regul Integr Comp Physiol 283: R553-R560.

8

ADRENOMEDULLIN AS AN ADIPOKINE

Kazuhiro Takahashi

Tohoku University School of Medicine, Sendai, Japan

INTRODUCTION

Obesity is one of the greatest and the most challenging problems in medicine of the 21st century, particularly in developed countries (Takahashi 2003). Adipocytes secrete a variety of bioactive substances, such as leptin (Zhang et al., 1994), adiponectin (Maeda et al., 1996), tumor necrosis factor-α (TNF-α) (Hotamisligil et al., 1993), and resistin (Steppan et al., 2001). These adipokines are thought to be related to the pathophysiology of various obesity-related diseases, such as type 2 diabetes mellitus, hypertension, stroke, and coronary heart diseases.

Adrenomedullin, originally isolated from pheochromocytoma (Kitamura et al., 1993), is produced and secreted by various types of cells, including neurons, glial cells, vascular smooth muscle and endothelial cells, cardiomyocytes, macrophages, fibroblasts and epithelial cells of various origins (Eto 2001; Takahashi 2001). Adrenomedullin has multiple biological functions, that are related not only to the vasodilator action, but also to the brain function, cell proliferation, cardiac function, hormone secretion, immune modulation, etc. Production and secretion of adrenomedullin by adipocytes, however, have not been studied until recently. We have shown that 3T3-L1 adipocytes express adrenomedullin (Li et al., 2003a; Li et al., 2003b). Expression of adrenomedullin in adipocytes or adipose tissues has recently been reported also by other investigators in abstract form (Fukai et al., 2003; Nambu et al., 2003). In this Chapter, the recent knowledge on adrenomedullin in adipocytes is summarized.

1. ADRENOMEDULLIN EXPRESSION DURING

ADIPOCYTE-DIFFERENTIATION IN 3T3-L1 CELLS

The 3T3-L1 cell line differentiates from preadipocytes to cells with morphological and biochemical properties of adipocytes by culturing under controlled conditions (Green et al., 1975; Green et al., 1976). In our study (Li et al., 2003a; Li et al., 2003b), 3T3-L1 cells were induced to differentiate to adipocytes by culturing in Dulbecco's modified Eagle's medium (DMEM) containing 10% fetal bovine serum (FBS), 1 μg/ml insulin, 1 μmol/l dexamethasone and 0.5 mmol/l 3-isobutyl-1-methylxanthine for 48 hours. The cells were then cultured in DMEM containing 10% FBS. Figure 1 shows Northern blot analysis of adrenomedullin mRNA during differentiation of 3T3-L1 cells. Adrenomedullin mRNA was detectable only in preadipocytes by Northern blot analysis. In contrast, resistin, an adipocyte-derived peptide hormone that was proposed to link obesity to insulin resistance and type 2 diabetes mellitus, was induced during differentiation to adipocytes.

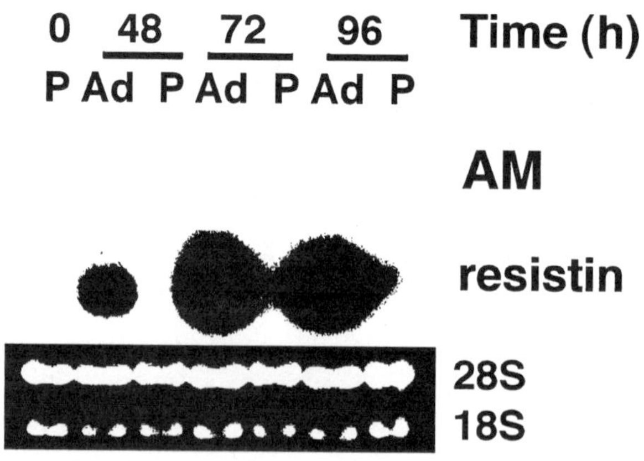

Figure 1. **Northern blot analysis of adrenomedullin and resistin mRNAs in 3T3-L1 adipocytes (Ad) and undifferentiated preadipocytes (P) harvested at 0, 48, 72, and 96h.** Each lane contains 15 μg total RNA. Lower panel: ethidium bromide staining of 28S and 18S ribosomal RNAs, showing even loading of total RNA in each lane. Reproduced from Li et al. Hypretension Res 2003; 26(Suppl):S41-S44, with kind permission from the Japanese Society of

Hypertension.

On the other hand, immunoreactive adrenomedullin was detected in the culture media of both 3T3-L1 preadipocytes and adipocytes by radioimmunoassay (Figure 2). Discrepant results between Northern blot analysis and radioimmunoassay may be due to higher sensitivity of radioimmunoassay. The concentrations of immunoreactive adrenomedullin in the culture medium of adipocytes were about 30% of preadipocytes. Thus, adrenomedullin expression is decreased during adipocyte-differentiation of 3T3-L1 cells. It is noteworthy, however, that 3T3-L1 adipocytes still has an ability to secrete adrenomedullin.

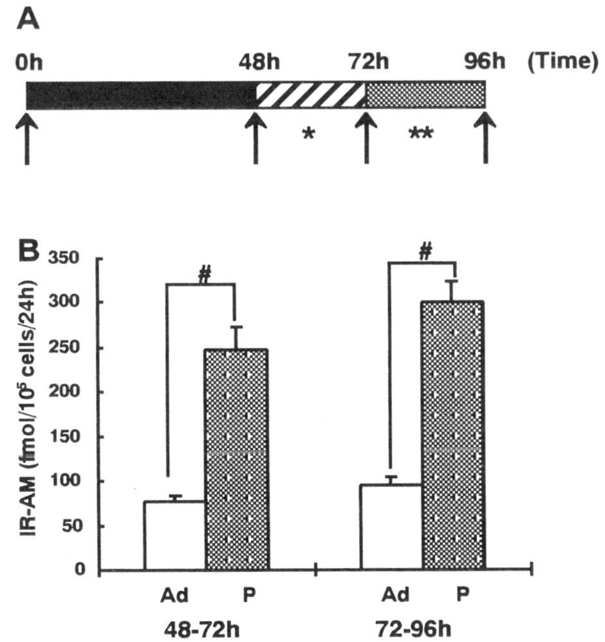

Figure 2. **Schematic presentation of the (A) experimental protocols and (B) immunoreactive-adrenomedullin (IR-AM) concentrations in the media of 3T3-L1 adipocytes (Ad) and undifferentiated preadipocytes (P).** 3T3-L1 cells were differentiated to adipocytes by culturing in medium containing 1 μg/ml insulin, 1 μmol/l dexamethasone and 0.5 mmol/l 3-isobutyl-1-methylxanthine (0-48 h) (shown

by a black bar). Conditioned media cultured for 48-72 h and 72-96 h were collected for the measurement of IR-AM (shown by * and **). Data are the mean±SEM (n=5). #P<0.0001. Cells were harvested for RNA extraction at 0, 48, 72, and 96h (shown by arrows). Resutlts in the RNA experiment are shown in Figure 1. Reproduced from Li et al. Hypretension Res 2003; 26(Suppl):S41-S44, with kind permission from the Japanese Society of Hypertension.

Fukai et al. have recently reported that expression of adrenomedullin was decreased in the early stage of adipocyte-differentiation, but was increased in the later stage of adipocyte-differentiation in 3T3-L1 cells (Fukai et al., 2003). We studied adrenomedullin expression in the early stage of adipocyte-differentiation of 3T3-L1 cells (Li et al., 2003a; Li et al., 2003b), and therefore can not deny the possibility that 3T3-L1 adipocytes with more maturation express adrenomedullin more abundantly.

2. TNF-α UPREGULATES ADRENOMEDULLIN EXPRESSION IN 3T3-L1 CELLS

TNF-α is secreted by adipocytes and supposed to be one of the major causes of insulin resistance in obese subjects (Hotamisligil et al., 1993). TNF-α antagonizes the stimulation of glucose uptake by insulin, and inhibits insulin-mediated tyrosine phosphorylation of the insulin receptor and insulin receptor substrate 1 (Feinstein et al., 1993; Hotamisligil et al., 1996). It also down-regulates glucose transporter GLUT4 gene expression (Stephens et al., 1991). To clarify whether TNF-α has a paracrine/autocrine effect on adrenomedullin secretion in adipocytes, we studied adrenomedullin expression in 3T3-L1 preadipocytes and adipocytes treated with TNF-α(Li et al., 2003b). Effects of two other cytokines, interferon-γ (IFN-γ) and interleukin-1β (IL-1β), on adrenomedullin expression were also studied. Treatment with TNF-α greatly augmented adrenomedullin mRNA expression levels in both preadipocytes and adipocytes (Figure 3). In preadipocytes, IL-1β slightly augmented adrenomedullin mRNA expression, whereas IFN-γ did not affect adrenomedullin mRNA expression. In adipocytes, either IL-1β or

IFN-γ had negligible effects on adrenomedullin mRNA expression. In contrast, TNF-α treatment inhibited resistin mRNA levels by about 60% compared with the untreated control in 3T3-L1 adipocytes.

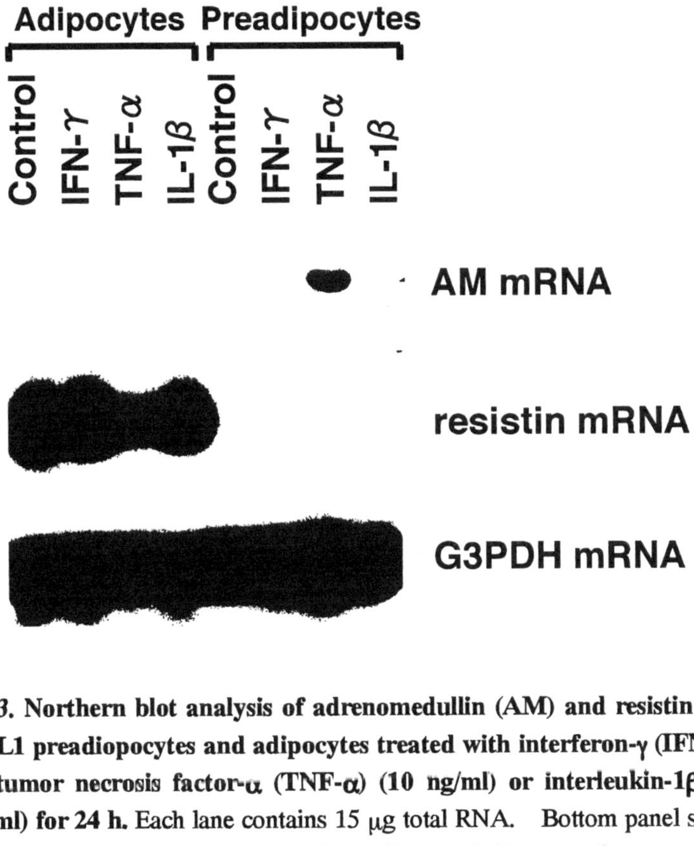

Figure 3. **Northern blot analysis of adrenomedullin (AM) and resistin mRNAs in 3T3-L1 preadiopocytes and adipocytes treated with interferon-γ (IFN-γ) (100 U/ml), tumor necrosis factor-α (TNF-α) (10 ng/ml) or interleukin-1β (IL-1β) (10 ng/ml) for 24 h.** Each lane contains 15 μg total RNA. Bottom panel shows the expression of G3PDH mRNA as an internal control. Data are from one of three independent experiments with similar results. Reproduced from Li et al. Eur J Endocrinol 2003; 149:231-238, with kind permission from the Society of the European Journal of Endocrinology.

Immunoreactive-adrenomedullin levels in the media were significantly elevated by 24 h treatment with 10 ng/ml TNF-α of both preadipocytes and adipocytes (Figure 4), and this elevation was more marked in preadipocytes than in adipocytes. IL-1β increased immunoreactive-adrenomedullin levels in the media of only preadipocytes. IFN-γ had no significant effects on immunoreactive-adrenomedullin levels in the media of either 3T3-L1 preadipocytes or adipocytes. Results in radioimmunoassay were mostly consistent with those in Northern blot analysis.

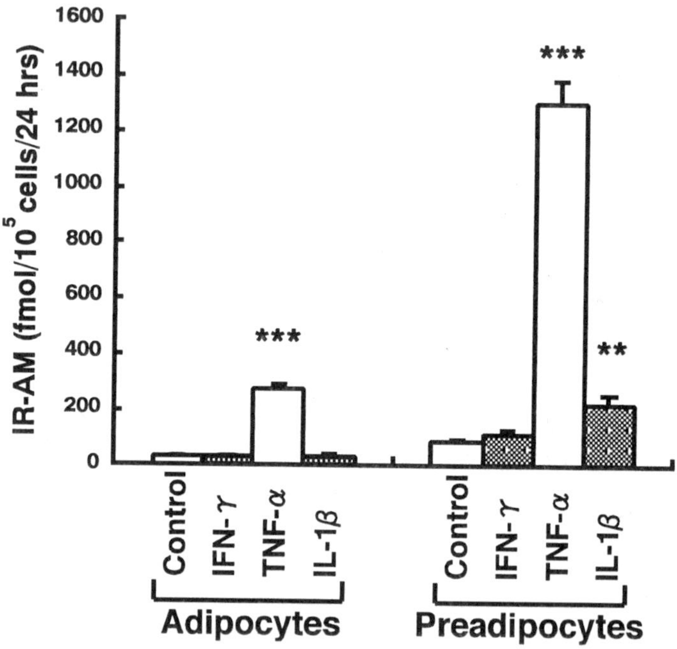

Figure 4. **Immunoreactive-adrenomedullin (IR-AM) in the medium of 3T3-L1 preadipocytes and adipocytes treated with interferon-γ (IFN-γ) (100 U/ml), tumor necrosis factor-α (TNF-α) (10 ng/ml) or interleukin-1β (IL-1β) (10 ng/ml) for 24 h.** Data are means ± S.E.M. (n=5). Statistical analysis was performed by one-way ANOVA followed by Fisher's protected least significant difference test. ** P<0.01, *** P<0.0001 (compared with untreated control within the same group). Reproduced from Li et al. Eur J Endocrinol 2003; 149:231-238, with kind permission from the Society of the European Journal of Endocrinology.

Reverse phase HPLC confirmed that the immunoreactive adrenomedullin in the media of TNF-α-treated and non-treated adipocytes consisted of mainly two immunoreactive peaks: a peak eluting in the position of authentic mouse adrenomedullin and a peak eluting in the position of mouse adrenomedullin with oxidized methionine (Figure 5). Material eluting in the position of mouse adrenomedullin with oxidized methionine may be generated during the culture or the extraction procedure. The peak eluting in the position of mouse adrenomedullin was greater in the medium obtained from 3T3-L1 adipocytes treated with TNF-α.

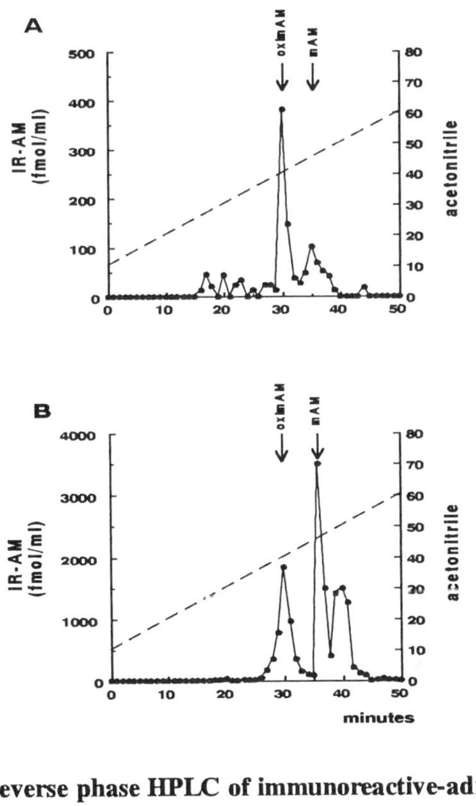

Figure 5. **Reverse phase HPLC of immunoreactive-adrenomedullin (IR-AM) in the medium of 3T3-L1 adipocytes.** (A) Without TNF-α treatment and (B) with TNF-α treatment (10 ng/ml) for 24 h. The arrows indicate the elution position of mouse AM (mAM) and mouse AM with oxidized methionine (oxi mAM). Dotted lines show a gradient of acetonitrile (%). Reproduced from Li et al. Eur J Endocrinol 2003; 149:231-238, with kind permission from the Society of the European Journal of Endocrinology.

Thus, adrenomedullin expression was induced by the treatment of TNF-α in both 3T3-L1 adipocytes and preadipocytes, similarly to the previous report in vascular smooth muscle cells by Sugo et al. (1994)

3. ADRENOMEDULLIN EXPRESSION IN ADIPOSE TISSUES

Nambu et al. reported high expression levels of adrenomedullin mRNA in the adipose tissue of mice, which were 2.2-9.6 times greater than those in kidney (Nambu et al., 2003). Adrenomedullin mRNA expression in human adipose tissue was about 70% of that in the human kidney. Furthermore, adrenomedullin mRNA was expressed more abundantly in the adipose tissues of genetically obese mice (*ob/ob* mice) than in control C57BL6 mice. The reason for discrepancy between their *in vivo* results (Nambu et al., 2003) and our results in 3T3-L1 adipocytes (Li et al., 2003a; Li et al., 2003b) remains to be determined. One possibility may be that some cytokines including TNF-α upregulate adrenomedullin expression in the adipose tissue *in vivo*. Another possibility may be that our findings in 3T3-L1 adipocytes may be related to the early differentiation to adipocytes, and that matured adipocytes express adrenomedullin more abundantly.

4. RECEPTORS AND BIOLOGICAL FUNCTIONS OF ADRENOMEDULLIN IN ADIPOCYTES

Adrenomedullin receptor consists of the complex of calcitonin-receptor-like receptor (CRLR) and receptor-activity modifying proteins (RAMPs) (McLatchie et al., 1998). There are at least three isoforms of RAMPs; RAMP1, 2, and 3. The RAMP1-CRLR complex generates the receptor specific for calcitonin gene-related peptide (CGRP) whereas the RAMP2-CRLR complex or the RAMP3-CRLR complex generates adrenomedullin-specific receptor. RAMP1, 2 and 3 are all expressed in the rat adipose tissue (Nagae et al., 2000). It is therefore plausible that adrenomedullin secreted from adipocytes acts on themselves as a paracrine or autocrine factor, possibly via the stimulation of the cyclic AMP pathway. The exact roles of adrenomedullin in adipocytes, however, remain to be determined. Funai et al. (2003) reported that adrenomedullin promotes adipocyte-differentiation.

It has recently been reported that adrenomedullin deficiency leads to insulin resistance using aged heterozygous adrenomedullin knockout mice (Shimosawa et al., 2003). Adrenomedullin has been shown to be an endogenous antioxidant that potently inhibits oxidative stress-induced vascular damage. Age-related overproduction of oxidative stress is also one of the causes of insulin resistance. Shimosawa et al. suggested that adrenomedullin is an endogenous substance counteracting oxidative stress-induced insulin resistance associated with aging. In this regard, it is tempting to speculate that decreased expression of adrenomedullin in adipocytes is related to a higher incidence of hypertension and type 2 diabetes mellitus in obese subjects.

Adrenomedullin is present in plasma and the plasma levels were elevated in patients with diabetes mellitus (Hayashi et al., 1997). Although Hayashi et al. speculated that elevated adrenomedullin in diabetes may originate from damaged vascular endothelial cells, it is possible that plasma adrenomedullin derives partly from adipocytes, in particular in obese subjects. Furthermore, adrenomedullin inhibits secretion of insulin from the pancreas (Martinez et al., 1996).

TNF-α is secreted by adipocytes and proposed to be a major cause for insulin resistance (Hotamisligil et al., 1993). TNF-α suppressed resistin expression and increased adrenomedullin expression in 3T3-L1 adipocytes, as shown in the previous section. The effects of TNF-α on expression of resistin and adrenomedullin therefore appear to be against insulin resistance.

SUMMARY

Adrenomedullin is expressed in cultured 3T3-L1 adipocytes and adipose tissues, and may act as a paracrine or autocrine factor. Adrenomedullin expression was decreased, however, during the adipocyte-differentiation of 3T3-L1 cells. Adrenomedullin expression is induced in 3T3-L1 adipocytes by TNF-α, a well-known mediator for insulin resistance. Although the physiological roles of adrenomedullin in adipocytes remain to be determined, the accumulating evidence suggests biological roles of adrenomedullin in the carbohydrate-lipid metabolism, and its pathophysiological roles in obesity-related diseases, such as type 2 diabetes mellitus and hypertension.

Acknowledgments: The author is grateful to Dr. Y. Li and Professor S. Shibahara for the collaboration of the present work. This work was supported in part by a Grant-in-aid for Scientific Research (B) from Japan Society for the Promotion of Science, by a Grant-in-aid for Scientific Research on Priority Areas (A) from the Ministry of Education, Culture, Sports, Science, and Technology of Japan, by a Research Grant from the HIROMI Medical Research Foundation (2001), by a Research Grant from the Intelligent Cosmos (2002 & 2003) and by the 21st Century COE program, Medical Science Center for Innovative Therapeutic Development Towards the Conquest of Signal Transduction Diseases.

REFERENCES

Eto T. (2001) A review of the biological properties and clinical implications of adrenomedullin and proadrenomedullin N-terminal 20 peptide (PAMP), hypotensive and vasodilating peptides. Peptides 22:1693-1711.

Feinstein R, Kanety H, Papa MZ, Lunenfeld B, and Karasik A. (1993) Tumor necrosis factor-alpha suppresses insulin-induced tyrosine phosphorylation of insulin receptor and its substrates. J Biol Chem 268:26055-26058.

Fukai N, Yoshimoto T, Sugiyama T, Ozawa N, Sato R, Shichiri M, Hirata Y. (2004) Concomitant expression of adrenomedullin and its receptor components in rat adipose tissues. Am J Physiol Endocrinol Metab (in press)

Green H and Kehinde O. (1975) An established preadipose cell line and its differentiation in culture. II. Factors affecting the adipose conversion. Cell 5:19-27.

Green H and Kehinde O. (1976) Spontaneous heritable changes leading to increased adipose conversion in 3T3 cells. Cell 7:105-113.

Hayashi M, Shimosawa T, Isaka M, Yamada S, Fujita R, and Fujita T. (1997) Plasma adrenomedullin in diabetes. Lancet 350:1449-1450.

Hotamisligil GS, Shargill NS, and Spiegelman BM. (1993) Adipose expression of tumor necrosis factor-alpha: direct role in obesity-linked insulin resistance. Science 259:87-91.

Hotamisligil GS, Peraldi P, Budavari A, Ellis R, White MF, and Spiegelman BM. (1996) IRS-1-mediated inhibition of insulin receptor tyrosine kinase activity in TNF-alpha- and obesity-induced insulin resistance. Science 271:665-8.

Kitamura K, Kangawa K, Kawamoto M, Ichiki Y, Nakamura S, Matsuo H, and Eto T. (1993a) Adrenomedullin: a novel hypotensive peptide isolated from human pheochromocytoma. Biochem Biophys Res Commun 192:553-560.

Li Y, Totsune K, Takeda K, Furuyama K, Shibahara S, and Takahashi K. (2003a) Decreased expression of adrenomedullin during adipocyte-differentiation of 3T3-L1 cells. Hypertens Res 26 (Suppl):S41-S44.

Li Y, Totsune K, Takeda K, Furuyama K, Shibahara S, and Takahashi K. (2003b) Differential expression of adrenomedullin and resistin in 3T3-L1 adipocytes treated with tumor necrosis factor-alpha. Eur J Endocrinol 149:231-238.

Maeda K, Okubo K, Shimomura I, Funahashi T, Matsuzawa Y, and Matsubara K. (1996) cDNA cloning and expression of a novel adipose specific collagen-like factor, apM1 (AdiPose Most abundant Gene transcript 1). Biochem Biophys Res Commun 221:286-289.

Martinez A, Weaver C, Lopez J, Bhathena SJ, Elsasser TH, Miller MJ, Moody TW, Unsworth EJ, and Cuttitta F. (1996) Regulation of insulin secretion and blood glucose metabolism by adrenomedullin. Endocrinology 137:2626-2632.

McLatchie LM, Fraser NJ, Main MJ, Wise A, Brown J, Thompson N, Solari R, Lee MG, and Foord SM. (1998) RAMPs regulate the transport and ligand specificity of the calcitonin-receptor-like receptor. Nature 393:333-339.

Nagae T, Mukoyama M, Sugawara A, Mori K, Yahata K, Kasahara M, Suganami T, Makino H, Fujinaga Y, Yoshioka T, Tanaka I, and Nakao K. (2000) Rat receptor-activity-modifying proteins (RAMPs) for adrenomedullin/CGRP receptor: cloning and upregulation in obstructive nephropathy. Biochem Biophys Res Commun 270:89-93.

Nambu T, Arai H, Moriyama K, Komatsu Y, and Nakao K. (2003) Adrenomedullin gene expression in adipose tissues. Program and Abstracts. The 7th Scientific Session of the Japanese Society of

Cardiovascular Endocrinology and Metabolism. p 94. (Abstract in Japanese)
Shimosawa T, Ogihara T, Matsui H, Asano T, Ando K, and Fujita T. (2003) Deficiency of adrenomedullin induces insulin resistance by increasing oxidative stress. Hypertension 41:1080-1085.
Stephens JM and Pekala PH. (1991) Transcriptional repression of the GLUT4 and C/EBP genes in 3T3-L1 adipocytes by tumor necrosis factor-alpha. J Biol Chem 266:21839-21845.
Steppan CM, Bailey ST, Bhat S, Brown EJ, Banerjee RR, Wright CM, Patel HR, Ahima RS, and Lazar MA. (2001) The hormone resistin links obesity to diabetes. Nature 409:307-312.
Sugo S, Minamino N, Shoji H, Kangawa K, Kitamura K, Eto T, and Matsuo H. (1994) Production and secretion of adrenomedullin from vascular smooth muscle cells: augmented production by tumor necrosis factor-alpha. Biochem Biophys Res Commun. 203:719-26.
Takahashi K. (2003) The brainstem is a key target for neuroendocrine research on obesity. Endocrinology 144:4690-4691. (Editorial)
Takahashi K. (2001) Adrenomedullin from a pheochromocytoma to the eye: implications of the adrenomedullin research for endocrinology in the 21st century. Tohoku J Exp Med 193:79-114.
Zhang Y, Proenca R, Maffei M, Barone M, Leopold L, and Friedman JM. (1994) Positional cloning of the mouse obese gene and its human homologue. Nature 372:425-432.

9

ADRENOMEDULLIN KNOCKOUT MOUSE AND TRANSGENIC MOUSE

Takayuki Shindo

Department of Cardiovascular Medicine, University of Tokyo, Tokyo, Japan

INTRODUCTION

Adrenomedullin (AM) is a vasodilating peptide involved in the regulation of circulatory homeostasis and in the pathophysiology of certain cardiovascular diseases. To elucidate the in vivo effects of AM, mice with manipulation of the AM gene have served as a useful tool for analysis of the physiological and pathophysiological functions of AM. Therefore, we established transgenic mice (AMTG) overexpressing AM and AM knockout mice (AMKO).

We established transgenic mice (AMTG) overexpressing AM driven by preproendothelin-1 (PPET-1) promoter. We constructed the transgene containing a 9.2-kb fragment of the murine PPET-1 gene 5'-flanking region including a 131-bp sequence of exon 1 and a 0.7-kb SV40-derived sequence with an intron and poly-A additional signal, between which AM cDNA was inserted. In this way, we gained AMTg overexpressing AM in a vessel-selective manner (Shindo et al., 2000).

Three independent groups including ours have reported the outcome of targeted AM gene disruption (Shindo et al., 2001; Caron et al., 2001; Shimosawa et al., 2002). Our strategy to knockout the AM gene was to substitute the neomycin resistance gene for the sequence encompassing exons 1 to 4. Heterozygote (AM+/-) were fully viable, and AM levels of the heart and lung of AM+/- lowered to half that of wild-type mice (WT). By contrast, mice homozygous for AM null mutation (AM-/-) were embryonic lethal, and no embryos could survive beyond the mid-term of gestation.

1. VASCULOGENESIS

The mortality rate among AM-/- embryos at E13.5 was 83%, and none survived to E14.5. The most apparent abnormality in AM-/- embryos at E13.5-14.0 was severe hemorrhage, which was observable under the skin and in the lung and liver. Hemorrhage was not yet detectable at E12.5-13.0, though the embryos showed abnormal vitelline vessels on the yolk sac (Figure 1); histological examination showed only the presence of poorly developed vitelline vessels, whereas the early stage of angiogenesis appeared to be normally processed. The umbilical artery was abnormally constricted. These embryos also exhibited accumulation of pericardial effusion suggestive of cardiac failure.

At E12.5, before hemorrhagic changes were detectable macroscopically, endothelial cells had partially detached from the basement structure in vessels. The endothelial cells in AM-/- embryos appeared cuboid in shape, rather than flat as in WT, and thus stood out from the wall of the lumen, leaving gaps where they were not adhering to the basement membrane (Figure 2). The three-layer structure of the basal membrane formed by the lamina rara interna, lamina densa and lamina rara externa was not clearly recognizable in AM-/- embryos. These changes may have contributed to the fragility of the vascular wall and subsequent hemorrhage.

These findings, together with the recent observation of the highly expressed AM in the placenta, fetal membrane, and amniotic fluid, indicate the indispensable roles of AM in the maintenance of circulatory homeostasis and vascular morphogenesis during fetal development.

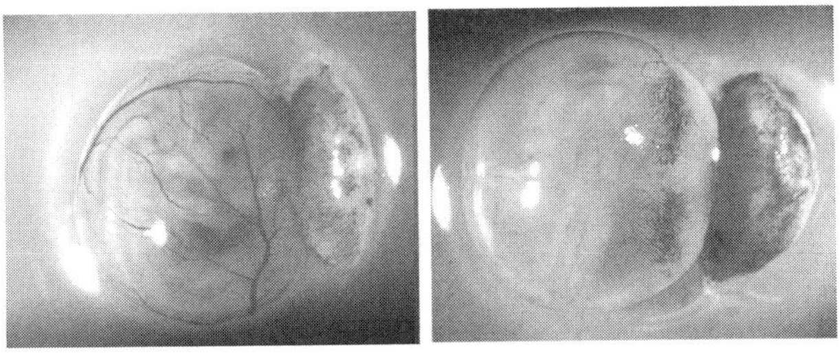

Figure 1. Appearance of E13.0 wild-type (left) and AM-/- (right) yolk sac. Well-developed vitelline vessels were detected on yolk sac of wild-type but were poorly developed in AM-/-.

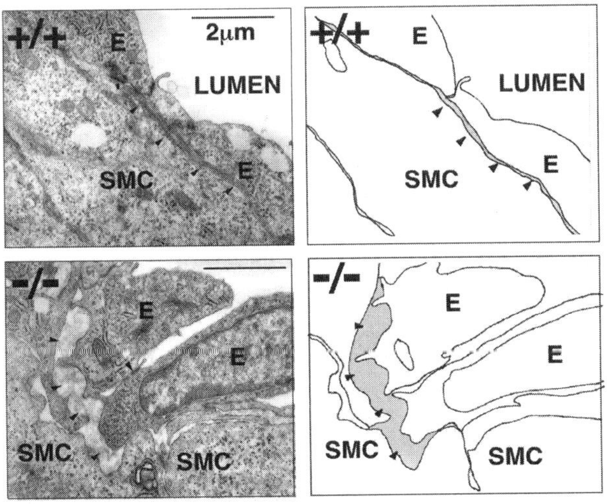

Figure 2. Transmission electron micrograph and schema of vascular structure from E12.5 wild-type (upper) and AM-/- (lower). E indicates endothelial cell. SMC indicates smooth muscle cell. Arrows indicate basement structure.

2. ARTERIOSCLEROSIS

We evaluated the effect of AM on neointimal hyperplasia and atherosclerosis using AMTG (Imai et al., 2002). We used cuff-injury model, in which a polyethylene tube cuff was placed around the femoral artery for 4 weeks. The area of neointima was significantly smaller in AMTG mice than in wild littermates (intima/media area ratio: AMTG 0.45+-0.14 vs WT 1.31+-0.41; $p<0.01$). The bromodeoxyuridine labeling index in the subendothelial layers, indicative of cell replication, was also significantly smaller in AMTG, indicating that proliferation of vascular smooth muscle cells was suppressed by AM overexpression. The vasculoprotective effect of AM was inhibited by chronic administration of N^G-nitro-L-arginine methyl ester (L-NAME), a nitric oxide (NO) synthase inhibitor, which suggests that this effect was at least partially mediated by NO. Moreover, we evaluated the effect of AM on atherosclerosis induced by hypercholesterolemia. We crossbred AMTG mice with ApoE knockout mice (ApoEKO) and fed the mice an atherogenic diet for 2 months. Atheromatous lesions were examined and showed significantly smaller in ApoEKO/AMTG than in ApoEKO (percent lesion area: ApoEKO/AMTG 12.0+-3.9 vs ApoEKO 15.8+-2.8%; $p<0.05$), although the lipid profiles before and after being fed an atherogenic diet were not affected by AM overexpression.
Collectively, AM has protective effects on injured or cholesterol-loaded vessels from neointima formation and atherosclerosis, suggesting that AM may have therapeutic potential in the treatment of atherosclerosis and vascular remodeling.

3. BLOOD PRESSURE REGULATION

In AMTG and AM+/-, we evaluated the hemodynamic parameters, including blood pressure and heart rate, by intraarterial cannulation

(Shindo et al., 2000; Shindo et al., 2001). Blood pressure was significantly lower in AMTG than in WT littermates (mean blood pressure: AMTG 109.3 +- 4.7 vs WT 124.4 +- 2.7 mm Hg). No significant change in heart rate accompanying the reduction in blood pressure was observed. To determine the extent to which the reduced blood pressure seen in AMTG was due to increased NO release, we studied the effects of N^G-monomethyl-L-arginine (L-NMMA), a NO synthase inhibitor, on blood pressure. The pressor response elicited by intravenous injection of L-NMMA was significantly higher in AMTG (AMTG 21.1 +- 3.3 vs WT 10.7 +- 1.3%; $p<0.01$); in fact, it offset the difference in blood pressure between the two groups. Plasma cGMP concentrations were significantly higher in AMTG than in WT mice, which is indicative of steady-state activation of the NO-cGMP pathway.

We also measured blood pressures in AM+/- mice and found them to be significantly higher than in WT (mean blood pressure: AM+/- 128.4 +- 2.2 vs WT 118.7 +-2.4 mm Hg).

We next examined the effects of acetylcholine (ACh), AM, and AM receptor antagonists AM(22-52) and CGRP(8-37) on the renal perfusion pressure (RPP) of kidneys isolated from AMTG, AM+/- and WT (Nishimatsu et al., 2002). Baseline RPP was significantly lower in AMTG than in AM+/-, and WT mice (AM+/- 93.4+-4.6, WT 85.8+-4.2, AMTG 72.4+-2.4 mm Hg, $p<0.01$). ACh and AM caused a dose-related reduction in RPP, but the degree of vasodilatation was smaller in AMTG than that in AM+/- and WT (% RPP 10^{-7}mol/L ACh: AM+/- 48.1+-3.9, WT 57.5+-5.6, AMTG 22.8+-4.8%, $p<0.01$). L-NAME caused greater vasoconstriction in AMTG (% RPP 10^{-4} mol/L L-NAME: AM+/- 33.1+-3.3, WT 55.5+-7.2, AMTG 152.6+-21.2%, $p<0.01$). Both AM antagonists increased RPP in AMTG to a greater extent compared with AM+/- and WT (% RPP 10^{-6}mol/L

CGRP(8-37): AM+/- 12.8+-2.6, WT 19.4+-3.6, AMTG 41.8+-8.7%, p<0.01).

We also evaluated the renal function and histology 24 hours after bilateral renal artery clamp for 45 minutes. In mice with ischemic kidneys, serum levels of urea nitrogen and renal damage scores showed smaller values in AMTG and greater values in AM+/- mice. However, the differences in serum urea nitrogen and renal damage scores among the 3 groups of mice were not observed in mice pretreated with L-NAME. Therefore, AM plays a role in the physiological regulation of the vascular tone and AM protects tissues from ischemia/reperfusion injury through its NO releasing activity.

Finally, our studies using transgenic and knockout mice demonstrated that AM has hypotensive and protective effects on organ and vasculature at postnatal stages as well as an important role in morphogenesis during the embyronic stage and in the maintenance of pregnancy. Further investigation is required on the underlying precise mechanisms of its diverse roles from embryo to adults.

REFERENCES

Caron KM, and Smithies O. (2001) Extreme hydrops fetalis and cardiovascular abnormalities in mice lacking a functional adrenomedullin gene. Proc Natl Acad Sci U S A.:98:615-619.

Imai Y, Shindo T, Maemura K, Sata M, Saito Y, Kurihara Y, Akishita M, Osuga J, Ishibashi S, Tobe K, Morita H, Oh-hashi Y, Suzuki T, Maekawa H, Kangawa K, Minamino N, Yazaki Y, Nagai R and Kurihara H. (2002) Resistance to neointimal hyperplasia and fatty streak formation in mice with adrenomedullin overexpression. Arterioscler Thromb Vasc Biol 22:1310-1315.

Nishimatsu H, Hirata Y, Shindo T, Kurihara H, Kakoki M, Nagata D, Hayakawa H, Satonaka H, Sata M, Tojo A, Suzuki E, Kangawa K, Matsuo H, Kitamura T and Nagai R. (2002) Role of endogenous adrenomedullin in the regulation of vascular tone and ischemic renal injury: studies on transgenic/knockout mice of adrenomedullin gene. Circ Res 90:657-663.

Shimosawa T, Shibagaki Y, Ishibashi K, Kitamura K, Kangawa K, Kato S, Ando K and Fujita T. (2002) Adrenomedullin, an endogenous peptide, counteracts cardiovascular damage. Circulation 105:106-111.

Shindo T, Kurihara H, Maemura K, Kurihara Y, Kuwaki T, Izumida T, Minamino N, Ju KH, Morita H, Oh-hashi Y, Kumada M, Kangawa K, Nagai R and Yazaki Y. (2000) Hypotension and resistance to lipopolysaccharide-induced shock in transgenic mice overexpressing adrenomedullin in their vasculature. Circulation 101:2309-2316.

Shindo T, Kurihara Y, Nishimatsu H, Moriyama N, Kakoki M, Wang Y, Imai Y, Ebihara A, Kuwaki T, Ju KH, Minamino N, Kangawa K, Ishikawa T, Fukuda M, Akimoto Y, Kawakami H, Imai T, Morita H, Yazaki Y, Nagai R, Hirata Y and Kurihara H. (2001) Vascular abnormalities and elevated blood pressure in mice lacking adrenomedullin gene. Circulation 104:1964-1971.

10

PLEIOTROPIC EFFECT OF ADRENOMEDULLIN: LESSONS FROM PURE ADRENOMEDULLIN KNOCKOUT MOUSE

Tatsuo Shimosawa, Katsuyuki Ando, and Toshiro Fujita

University of Tokyo, Faculty of Medicine, Tokyo, Japan

INTRODUCTION

AM shares the same precursor, proadrenomedullin, with proadrenomedullin N-terminal 20 peptide (PAMP) (Kitamura et al., 1994) a compound showing physiological effects different from those of AM (Shimosawa et al., 1995; Shimosawa et al., 1996; Shimosawa et al., 1997). Several studies revealed that AM is a multipotent peptide (Kusaka et al., 1996; Ando et al., 1998; Taylor et al., 2001; Kawai et al., 2002) and a new tool for use in diagnosis of extracellular volume in renal insufficiency (Kanozawa et al., 2002). However, as is other vasoactive peptides, technical limitations have restricted the study of the physiological relevance of AM and PAMP. To overcome these limitations, gene manipulations were done and it revealed pleiotropic effects of AM.

Generating AM/PAMP transgenic mice and knockout mice

As mentioned above, AM and PAMP share the same propeptide and signal peptide and thus they are encoded on one gene. This construction made it difficult to separate AM transgene from PAMP transgene. Our preliminary studies showed that direct conjugation of original signal peptide and AM peptide sequence was not sufficient for various cells to secrete AM. Therefore, gene delivery models (Chao et al., 1997; Dobrzynski et al., 2000; Zhang et al., 2000; Wang et al., 2001) and AM transgenic mice (Shindo et al., 2000) induced both AM and PAMP at the same time. The transgenic mice were applied endothelin promoter to express AM/PAMP only in endothelial cells. And it showed that AM can protect organs from septic shock (Shindo et al., 2000) or high fat diet (Imai et al., 2002) possibly by increasing NO synthesis (Nishimatsu et al., 2002).

As for disruption of AM, gene knockout and ribozyme methods have been reported. Three independent groups reported AM or AM/PAMP knockout mice (Caron et al., 2001; Shindo et al., 2001; Shimosawa et al., 2002). Two groups generated AM/PAMP knockout mice by replacing one exon with NEO resistant gene (Caron et al., 2001; Shindo et al., 2001) and we generate AM knockout mice by inserting stop mutation at the beginning of AM coding region (Shimosawa et al., 2002). This AM knockout mice revealed not to affect the expression of PAMP and PAMP was secreted to the same extent with wild type (Shimosawa et al., 2002).

AM knockout mice are embryonic lethal and thus there remained limitation of study, Taylor et al. applied ribozyme to block AM synthesis genetically (Taylor et al., 2002). They showed that AM disruption led to an exaggerated drinking response in rats.

1. Fetus growth

AM/PAMP knockout mice and AM knockout mice revealed embryonic lethal(Caron et al., 2001; Shindo et al., 2001; Shimosawa et al., 2003a). The cause of the lethality varies from report to report.

Caron et al. reported that AM/PAMP knockout mice are hydrops fetalis and they assumed that lymphatic circulation plays a role in lethality (Caron et al., 2001). On the other hand, Shindo et al. reported poor vascular formation in yolk sac and fetus showed massive hemorrhage with abnormal basement membrane of vessels (Shindo et al., 2001). AM knockout mice are also embryonic lethal, however, no hydrops fetalis or hemorrhage were found and histological examination throughout the body showed no apparent abnormalities in homozygotes (Shimosawa et al., 2003a). So far the precise mechanism of its lethality is still unclear, however, exogenous supplementation of AM failed rescue fetus, AM effect in gestation should be highly essential.

2. Regulation of blood flow and organ protection

Gene delivery to spontaneously hypertensive rats, DOCA-salt rats or Dahl salt-sensitive rats revealed that AM decreased blood pressure concomitant with increased cAMP level. In line with decreases in blood pressure, renal and cardiovascular damage were attenuated (Chao et al., 1997; Dobrzynski et al., 2000; Zhang et al., 2000; Wang et al., 2001). It is suggested that direct vasodilatory action of AM plays a key role in organ protection from hypertension.

Besides direct action, there are reports that AM protects organs from several stress by indirect fashion. In ischemic heart model (Kato et al., 2003), pulmonary hypertension model (Yoshihara et al., 1998; Nagaya et al., 2003b), AM could protect organs from damage by inhibiting apoptosis or cell proliferations. Also, ischemic damages in kidney were protected in AM transgenic mice and deteriorated in AM/PAMP knockout mice (Nishimatsu et al., 2002) by inducing NO synthesis. Septic shock model of AM transgenic mice revealed that

AM preserves liver function after septic shock by producing NO (Shindo et al., 2001). From these observations, it is speculated that AM protects organs by preserving blood flow via increasing NO synthesis. This speculation is supported studies which revealed that inhibition of guanylate cyclase attenuated AM-induced vasodilation in rat aorta (Hayakawa et al., 1999) or blockade of NO synthesis attenuated AM-induced increases of renal blood flow (Hirata et al., 1995).

3. Antioxidant effect and organ protection

Recent studies showed that oxidative stress is one cause of organ damage in variety of pathological condition. Specially, ischemia-reperfusion, hypertension, or diabetic condition increases oxidative stress and induces vascular damage, renal damage or other organ damages. AM expression is increased by oxidative stress (Ando et al., 1998; Chun et al., 2000). At the same time, AM inhibits oxidative stress formation (Chini et al., 1997). These observation leads us to hypothesize that AM is an intrinsic antioxidants. To clarify this hypothesis, we administered angiotensin II and salt diet which was known to increase oxidative stress. By this manipulation, we showed that AM knockout mice had higher oxidative stress in three ways; urinary excretion of oxidative stress markers such as isoprostane and 8-OHdG, immunostaining of 3-nitrotyrosine to localize oxidative stress and real time oxidant production measurement by electron spin resonance method (Shimosawa et al., 2002). Moreover, the increased oxidative stress was reduced by supplementation of AM. The blood pressure was comparable between wild type and AM deficient mice, but the fibrotic changes and occlusion of coronary artery were more apparent in AM deficient mice than in wild type. This change was reversed by 4-hydroxyTEMPO, a superoxide dismutase mimetic (Noiri et al., 2001). From this study, it was revealed that AM was an organ protective peptide by inhibiting oxidative stress.

In hypoxia model or cuff-induced vascular damage model, it also revealed that AM is an endogenous antioxidant and when it is used topically, it can reverse vascular damages (Kawai et al., 2004; Matsui et al., in press).

Ageing is also well known to accumulate oxidative stress and cause age-related diseases. Aged AM knockout mice also accumulate larger amount of oxidative stress than wild-type mice. We observed aged AM knockout mice are insulin-resistant and it is reversed by SOD mimetics or AM administration (Shimosawa et al., 2003b).

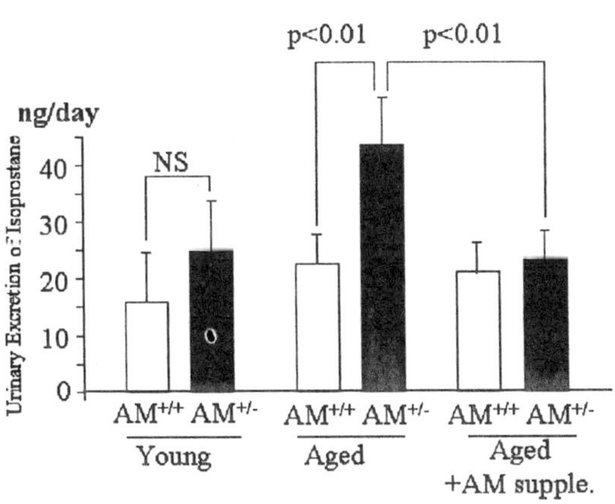

Fig. 1. Oxidative stress in aged AM knockout mice and therapeutical potency of AM. Oxidative stress was monitored by urinary excretion of 8-isoprostane.

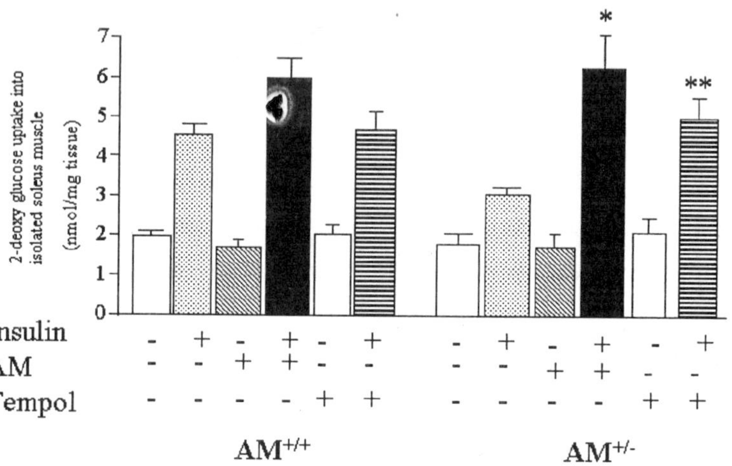

Fig. 2. Insulin resistance in aged AM knockout mice. Insulin resistance are measured by insulin-stimulated glucose uptake to soleus muscle. Tempol; an membrane permeable SOD mimetics. *, and **; p<0.01 vs. AM+/- with neither AM supplementation nor tempol treatment

FUTURE DIRECTION AND CONCLUSION

Because of the embryonic lethality in AM and PAMP, knockout mice, there remains limitation to clarify the physiological and pathological role of AM and PAMP. However, from studies using heterozygote, pleiotropic effects of AM has been clarified and its therapeutical potency are expected. Indeed, based upon these data and pharmacological data, clinical trial of AM in pulmonary hypertensives is reported (Nagaya et al., 2003a) and it is very promising. As for PAMP, we still do not have specific receptors and we have to wait. In contrast, we can generate PAMP transgenic mice. A few studies showed that PAMP modifies sympathetic nerve tone and regulate blood pressure (Shimosawa et al., 1997). The physiological effect is totally different from that of AM and PAMP transgenic mice has potential to reveal new aspects in both therapeutical and diagnosis.

REFERENCES

Ando K., Ito Y., Kumada M. and Fujita T. (1998). Oxidative stress increases adrenomedullin mRNA levels in cultured rat vascular smooth muscle cells. Hypertens Res 21: 187-91.

Caron K. M. and Smithies O. (2001). Extreme hydrops fetalis and cardiovascular abnormalities in mice lacking a functional Adrenomedullin gene. Proc Natl Acad Sci U S A 98: 615-619.

Chao J., Jin L., Lin K. F. and Chao L. (1997). Adrenomedullin gene delivery reduces blood pressure in spontaneously hypertensive rats. Hypertens Res 20: 269-77.

Chini E., Chini C., Bolliger C., Jougasaki M., Grande J., Burnett J. J. and Dousa T. (1997). Cytoprotective effects of adrenomedullin in glomerular cell injury: central role of cAMP signaling pathway. Kidney Int 52: 917-925.

Chun T., Itoh H., Saito T., Yamahara K., Doi K., Mori Y., Ogawa Y., Yamashita J., Tanaka T., Inoue M., Masatsugu K., Sawada N., Fukunaga Y. and Nakao K. (2000). Oxidative stress augments secretion of endothelium-derived relaxing peptides, C-type natriuretic peptide and adrenomedullin. J Hypertens 18: 575-580.

Dobrzynski E., Wang C., Chao J. and Chao L. (2000). Adrenomedullin gene delivery attenuates hypertension, cardiac remodeling, and renal injury in deoxycorticosterone acetate-salt hypertensive rats. Hypertension 36: 995-1001.

Hayakawa H., Hirata Y., Kakoki M., Suzuki Y., Nishimatsu H., Nagata D., Suzuki E., Kikuchi K., Nagano T., Kangawa K., Matsuo H., Sugimoto T. and Omata M. (1999). Role of nitric oxide-cGMP pathway in adrenomedullin-induced vasodilation in the rat. Hypertension 33: 689-93.

Hirata Y., Hayakawa H., Suzuki Y., Suzuki E., Ikenouchi H., Kohmoto O., Kimura K., Kitamura K., Eto T., Kangawa K., Matsuo H. and Omata M. (1995). Mechanisms of adrenomedullin-induced vasodilation in the rat kidney. Hypertension 25: 790-795.

Imai Y., Shindo T., Maemura K., Sata M., Saito Y., Kurihara Y., Akishita M., Osuga J., Ishibashi S., Tobe K., Morita H., Oh-hashi Y., Suzuki T., Maekawa H., Kangawa K., Minamino N., Yazaki Y., Nagai R., Kurihara H., Nishimatsu H., Hirata Y., Kakoki M., Nagata D., Hayakawa H., Satonaka H., Tojo A., Suzuki E., Matsuo H. and Kitamura T. (2002). Resistance to neointimal hyperplasia and fatty streak formation in mice with adrenomedullin overexpression

Role of endogenous adrenomedullin in the regulation of vascular tone and ischemic renal injury: studies on transgenic/knockout mice of adrenomedullin gene. Arterioscler Thromb Vasc Biol 22: 1310-5.

Kanozawa K., Shimosawa T., Nagasawa R., Matsuda A., Kato H., Matsumura O., Mitarai T., Isoda K. and Fujita T. (2002). Mature form of adrenomedullin is a useful marker to evaluate blood volume in hemodialysis patients. Am J Kid Dis 40: 794-801.

Kato K., Yin H., Agata J., Yoshida H., Chao L. and Chao J. (2003). Adrenomedullin Gene Delivery Attenuates Myocardial Infarction and Apoptosis after Ischemia and Reperfusion. Am J Physiol Heart Circ Physiol 12: 12.

Kawai J., Ando K., Shimosawa T., Harii K. and Fujita T. (2002). Regional hemodynamic effects of adrenomedullin in Wistar rats: a comparison with calcitonin gene-related peptide. Hypertens Res 25: 441-446.

Kawai J., Ando K., Tojo A., Shimosawa T., Takahashi K., Onozato M., Yamasaki M., Ogita T., Nakaoka T. and Fujita T. (2004). Endogenous Adrenomedullin Protects against Vascular Response to Injury in Mice. Circulation 109: 1147-1153.

Kitamura K., Kangawa K., Ishiyama Y., Washimine H., Ichiki Y., Kawamoto M., Minamino N., Matsuo H. and Eto T. (1994). Identification and hypotensive activity of proadrenomedullin N-terminal 20 peptide (PAMP). FEBS Letters 351: 35-37.

Kusaka I., Ishikawa S., Fujita N., Higashiyama M., Honda K., Okada K. and Saito T. (1996). Inhibition by adrenomedullin of arginine vasopressin-activated mitogen-activated protein kinase in rat glomerular mesangial cells via cAMP production. Hypertens Res 19: 113-9.

Matsui H., Shimosawa T., Itakura K., Xing G., Ando K. and Fujita T. (in press). Adrenomedullin can protect against pulmonary vascular remodeling induced by hypoxia. Circulation.

Nagaya N., Miyatake K., Kyotani S., Nishikimi T., Nakanishi N. and Kangawa K. (2003a). Pulmonary vasodilator response to adrenomedullin in patients with pulmonary hypertension. Hypertens Res 26: S141-6.

Nagaya N., Okumura H., Uematsu M., Shimizu W., Ono F., Shirai M., Mori H., Miyatake K. and Kangawa K. (2003b). Repeated inhalation of adrenomedullin ameliorates pulmonary hypertension and survival in monocrotaline rats. Am J Physiol Heart Circ Physiol 285: H2125-31.

Nishimatsu H., Hirata Y., Shindo T., Kurihara H., Kakoki M., Nagata D., Hayakawa H., Satonaka H., Sata M., Tojo A., Suzuki E., Kangawa K., Matsuo H., Kitamura T. and Nagai R. (2002). Role of endogenous adrenomedullin in the regulation of vascular tone and ischemic renal injury: studies on transgenic/knockout mice of adrenomedullin gene.

Circ Res 90: 657-63.

Noiri E., Nakao A., Uchida K., Tsukahara H., Ohno M., Fujita T., Brodsky S. and Goligorsky M. S. (2001). Oxidative and nitrosative stress in acute renal ischemia. Am J Physiol Renal Physiol 281: F948-57.

Shimosawa T., Ando K. and Fujita T. (1997). Newly identified peptide, proadrenomedullin N-terminal 20 peptide induces hypotensive action via pertussis toxin-sensitive G-proteins. Hypertension 30: 1009-1014.

Shimosawa T. and Fujita T. (1996). Hypotensive effect of newly identified peptide, proadrenomedullin N-terminal 20 peptide. Hypertension 28: 325-329.

Shimosawa T., Ito Y., Ando K., Kitamura K., Kangawa K. and Fujita T. (1995). Proadrenomedullin NH2 -terminal 20 peptide, a new product of the adrenomedullin gene, inhibits norepinephrine overflow from nerve endings. J Clin Invest 96: 1672-1676.

Shimosawa T., Matsui H., Xing G., Itakura K., Ando K. and Fujita T. (2003a). Organ-protective effects of adrenomedullin. Hypertens Res 26: S109-12.

Shimosawa T., Ogihara T., Matsui H., Asano T., Ando K. and Fujita T. (2003b). Deficiency of adrenomedullin induces insulin resistance by increasing oxidative stress. Hypertension 41: 1080-1085.

Shimosawa T., Shibagaki Y., Ishibashi K., Kitamura K., Kangawa K., Kato S., Ando K. and Fujita T. (2002). Adrenomedullin, an Endogenous Peptide, Counteracts Cardiovascular Damage. Circulation 105: 106-111.

Shindo T., Kurihara H., Maemura K., Kurihara Y., Kuwaki T., Izumida T., Minamino N., Ju K. H., Morita H., Oh-hashi Y., Kumada M., Kangawa K., Nagai R. and Yazaki Y. (2000). Hypotension and resistance to lipopolysaccharide-induced shock in transgenic mice overexpressing adrenomedullin in their vasculature. Circulation 101: 2309-16.

Shindo T., Kurihara Y., Nishimatsu H., Moriyama N., Kakoki M., Wang Y., Imai Y., Ebihara A., Kuwaki T., Ju K. H., Minamino N., Kangawa K., Ishikawa T., Fukuda M., Akimoto Y., Kawakami H., Imai T., Morita H., Yazaki Y., Nagai R., Hirata Y. and Kurihara H. (2001). Vascular abnormalities and elevated blood pressure in mice lacking adrenomedullin gene. Circulation 104: 1964-71.

Taylor M., Shimosawa T. and Samson W. (2001). Endocrine and metabolic action of adrenomedullin. The Endocrinologist 11: 171-177.

Taylor M. M. and Samson W. K. (2002). Ribozyme compromise of adrenomedullin mRNA reveals a physiological role in the regulation of water intake. Am J Physiol Regul Integr Comp Physiol 282: R1739-45.

Wang C., Dobrzynski E., Chao J. and Chao L. (2001). Adrenomedullin gene delivery attenuates renal damage and cardiac hypertrophy in Goldblatt hypertensive rats. Am J Physiol Renal Physiol 280: F964-71.

Yoshihara F., Nishikimi T., Horio T., Yutani C., Takishita S., Matsuo H., Ohe T. and Kangawa K. (1998). Chronic infusion of adrenomedullin reduces pulmonary hypertension and lessens right ventricular hypertrophy in rats administered monocrotaline. Eur J Pharmacol 355: 33-9.

Zhang J. J., Yoshida H., Chao L. and Chao J. (2000). Human adrenomedullin gene delivery protects against cardiac hypertrophy, fibrosis, and renal damage in hypertensive dahl salt-sensitive rats. Hum Gene Ther 11: 1817-27.

11

THERAPEUTIC APPLICATION OF ADRENOMEDULLIN

Toshio Nishikimi[1], Noritoshi Nagaya[2], Kenji Kangawa[2], Hiroaki Matsuoka[1]

[1]*Department of Hypertension and Cardiorenal Medicine, Dokkyo University Medical School, Tochigi, Japan and* [2]*National Cardiovascular Center Research Institute, Osaka, Japan*

INTRODUCTION

Intravenous infusion of adrenomedullin (AM) causes potent and sustained hypotension in animals and humans, (Kitamura et al., 1993; Parks et al., 1997; Nakamura et al., 1997) and its effect is comparable to that of CGRP (Kitamura et al., 1993). Acute administration of AM reduces total peripheral resistance and decreases blood pressure. This is concomitant with a rise in heart rate, cardiac output, and stroke volume (Ishiyama et al, 1993). Similar effects are seen in conscious rats (Gardiner et al, 1995).

Renal effects of AM have been reported. Ebara et al. (Ebara et al., 1994) reported that acute administration of AM into the renal artery had no effect on heart rate or mean arterial pressure, but increased renal blood flow, urine output, and urinary sodium excretion in a dose-dependent manner, indicative of a direct vasodilatory effect on preglomerular and postglomerular arterioles. Subsequent studies revealed that this effect is mediated partly via an endothelial, NO-dependent mechanism (Miura et al., 1995; Hirata et al., 1995). These results suggest that increased plasma and renal produced AM may affect renal function, and evidence exists for a role for locally produced AM in tubular function (Nishikimi et al., 2001).

Endocrine effect of AM also has been reported. Yamaguchi et al (Yamaguchi et al., 1995) reported that AM significantly inhibited aldosterone secretion in response to angiotensin II, K^+, and the calcium ionophore A23187 from dispersed rat adrenal zona glomerulosa cells. The same group (Yamaguchi et al, 1996) studied the effect of AM on aldosterone production. They showed that AM administration significantly inhibited aldosterone production, but had no effect on adrenal or renin, plasma corticosterone, or K^+ levels.
Thus, multiple effects of AM on hemodynamic, renal, and endocrine system indicate that administration of AM may be effective in the treatment of cardiovascular diseases such as heart failure, hypertension, renal failure, and pulmonary hypertension.

1. ACUTE ADMINISTRATION OF AM

(1) Heart Failure

Rademaker et al. (Rademaker et al., 1997) first reported that acute administration of AM increased plasma cAMP levels in association with dose-dependent falls in calculated peripheral resistance, mean arterial pressure, and left atrial pressure and increases in cardiac output in sheep with pacing-induced heart failure. They showed that AM increased urinary sodium excretion, creatinine and cAMP excretion, and creatinine clearance with a reduction of plasma aldosterone levels. We also examined the cardiovascular and renal effects of two doses of intravenous infusion of AM in rats with heart failure (Nagaya et al., 1999). Low-dose AM increased urine flow and urinary sodium excretion without changes in any hemodynamic variables. In contrast, high-dose AM slightly decreased mean arterial pressure and significantly increased cardiac output in heart failure and normal rats. Infusion of high-dose AM also resulted in significant decreases in right ventricular systolic pressure and right atrial pressure only in heart failure rats. High-dose AM significantly increased glomerular filtration rate and renal plasma flow as well as urine flow and urinary sodium excretion. These studies imply an important pathophysiological role for AM in the regulation of pressure and volume in heart failure and raise the possibility of a new therapeutic approach to this disease.

Indeed, we examined the effect of intravenous administration of AM on hemodynamic, renal, and hormonal responses in patients with heart failure (Nagaya et al., 2000). AM markedly increased cardiac index while decreasing pulmonary capillary wedge pressure in heart failure and normal subjects. AM significantly decreased mean pulmonary arterial pressure only in heart failure subjects and AM increased urine volume and urinary sodium excretion in both groups. Plasma aldosterone significantly decreased during and after AM infusion only in heart failure. These results indicate that intravenous infusion of AM has beneficial hemodynamic, renal, and hormonal effects in patients with heart failure. Lainchbury et al. (Lainchbury et al., 1999) also reported that AM and brain natriuretic peptide, at plasma concentrations within the pathophysiological range, have beneficial hemodynamic, renal, and hormonal effects in patients with heart failure. The same group recently reported that the effect of coadministration of AM and endopeptidase inhibitor in sheep with heart failure, because AM is considered to be metabolized in part by neutral endopeptidase (Rademaker et al., 2002a). Coadministration of AM and endopeptidase inhibitor produced hemodynamic effects greater than those achieved during administration of AM alone. Despite the larger falls in blood pressure, renal function was improved and elevations in plasma AM and cAMP were greater than those during administration of AM alone. These results suggest that cotreatment with AM and an endopeptidase inhibitor has beneficial hemodynamic and renal effects in heart failure. Thus, the combination therapy of AM and endopeptidase inhibitor may be one possible approach for the treatment of heart failure (see Chapter 12 in detail).

(2) Hypertension and Chronic Renal Failure

Troughton et al. (Troughton et al., 2000) examined the effects of the intravenous infusion of AM in subjects with essential hypertension. They used intravenous AM at a low and a high dose (2.9 and 5.8 pmol/kg/min). Plasma AM reached pathophysiological levels during infusion, with a concurrent rise in plasma cAMP. High-dose AM increased peak heart rate, lowered systolic and diastolic blood pressure, and increased cardiac output. Despite a rise in plasma renin activity during high-dose AM, aldosterone levels were not altered. Plasma norepinephrine and epinephrine levels increased with high-dose AM. AM had no significant effect on urine volume or sodium excretion.

The same group also studied the effects of AM infusion at high dose and low dose (2.9 and 5.8 pmol/kg/min) in subjects with chronic renal impairment (McGregor et al, 2002). AM infusion achieved plasma AM concentrations in the pathophysiological range after the low- and high-dose infusion. Compared with the vehicle control, high-dose AM increased peak heart rate and cardiac output and lowered both systolic and diastolic blood pressures. Plasma renin activity, angiotensin II, and norepinephrine increased by up to 50% above baseline levels, whereas aldosterone and epinephrine were unchanged. Urinary volume and sodium excretion increased significantly with low-dose AM, whereas creatinine clearance was stable, and proteinuria tended to decrease. Thus, AM may have a role in modulating blood pressure and kidney function in renal disease.

(3) Pulmonary Hypertension

Nagaya et al. (Nagaya et al., 2000a) investigated the effects of intravenous infusion of AM in patients with pulmonary hypertension. They measured the hemodynamic and hormonal responses to intravenous infusion of AM in patients with precapillary pulmonary hypertension. Infusion of AM produced a 44% increase in cardiac index and a 32% decrease in pulmonary vascular resistance, without a significant change in mean pulmonary arterial pressure. AM also decreased mean systemic arterial pressure and increased heart rate. AM decreased plasma aldosterone without causing a significant change in plasma renin activity. Plasma atrial and brain natriuretic peptides tended to decrease with AM, although these changes did not reach the levels of significance. Thus, intravenous AM has beneficial hemodynamic and hormonal effects in patients with precapillary pulmonary hypertension (see chapter 12 in detail).

2. CHRONIC ADMINISTRATION OF AM

(1) Hypertension

There have been few reports which investigated the effect of chronic administration of AM in cardiovascular disease. Khan et al. (Khan et al., 1997a) reported that chronically infused human AM (200 ng/h, for 2 weeks) had a hypotensive effect in both normotensive rats and spontaneously hypertensive rats without an increase in urinary volume or sodium excretion at a plasma AM concentration within the physiological limit. The same investigators also demonstrated that chronically infused AM (1000 ng/h, for 2 weeks) had a hypotensive effect accompanied by significant reductions of plasma renin activity and plasma aldosterone concentration in renovascular hypertensive rats at a plasma AM concentration within the physiological rang (Khan et al., 1997b). These results imply that chronic AM infusion may have beneficial effects in hypertension and its organ damage in part via inhibition of the renin-angiotensin system.

We reported that chronic human AM infusion (500 ng/h) has renoprotective effects in a rat model of malignant hypertension (Nishikimi et al., 2002; Mori et al., 2002). AM infusion significantly reduced plasma renin concentration, plasma aldosterone levels and plasma endogenous rat AM levels within the physiological range of human plasma AM levels. AM decreased urinary protein excretion and improved glomerular sclerosis, according to the histological findings. AM significantly decreased the intrarenal angiotensin II levels and gene expression of TGF-beta and angiotensin converting enzyme. These results suggest that increased endogenous AM plays a compensatory role in chronic hypertensive renal failure and that long-term AM infusion has renoprotective effects in this type of hypertension model, partly via inhibition of the circulating and renal renin-angiotensin system.

(2) Heart Failure

Plasma AM levels are increased in heart failure, and acute administration of AM exerts beneficial hemodynamic, renal, and neurohormonal effects in heart failure. However, the chronic effects of AM administration on heart failure remain unknown. Rademaker et al. (Rademaker et al., 2002b) infused AM (10 ng/kg per minute) for 4 days in sheep with pacing-induced heart failure. Infusion of AM persistently increased circulating levels of the AM, in association with prompt (15 minutes) and sustained (4 days) increases in cardiac output (day 4, 27%), and reductions in peripheral resistance (30%), mean arterial pressure (13%), and left atrial pressure (24%). AM also significantly enhanced urinary sodium excretion (day 4, 3-fold), creatinine excretion (1.2-fold), and creatinine clearance (1.4-fold) over the 4 days of treatment, whereas urine volume and cAMP excretion tended to be elevated. These findings support the concept of AM as a protective hormone during hemodynamic compromise with therapeutic potential in heart failure.

We examined the effect of chronic infusion of AM (500 ng/min, for 7 weeks) on the progression of heart failure in Dahl salt-sensitive rats (Nishikimi et al., 2003). Chronic AM infusion significantly decreased left ventricular end-diastolic pressure, right ventricular systolic pressure, right atrial pressure, and left ventricular weight/body weight. AM significantly attenuated the increase in circulating renin-aldosterone, endogenous rat AM, and atrial natriuretic peptide levels. AM also decreased the myocardial tissue levels of angiotensin II and atrial and brain natriuretic peptide. These changes were associated with the improvement of cardiac output and systemic vascular resistance. Furthermore, AM improved left ventricular end-systolic elastance. These improvements were greater in the AM than in the diuretic group, although both drugs similarly decreased systolic blood pressure and increased urinary sodium excretion. Kaplan-Meier survival analysis showed that AM significantly prolonged survival time compared with those of the diuretic and vehicle treatment groups. These results suggest that endogenous AM plays a compensatory role in heart failure and that chronic AM infusion attenuates progression of left ventricular dysfunction and improves survival, at least in part, through inhibition of circulating and myocardial neurohormonal activation.

(3) Myocardial Infarction

Nakamura et al. (Nakamura et al., 2002) examined the effects of long-term administration of AM on left ventricular remodeling following acute myocardial infarction. They infused human recombinant AM for 4 weeks in rats with myocardial infarction induced by left coronary artery ligation. Chronic infusion of AM reduced the heart weight/body weight, left ventricular end-diastolic pressure, plasma endogenous rat AM levels, myocyte size, and collagen volume fraction of non-infarct LV area without affecting the infarct size, indicating that continuous administration of AM could be a useful therapeutic tool for acute MI.

Okumura et al. (Okumura et al., 2004) recently examined the effect of infusion of AM on myocardial ischemia/reperfusion following acute myocardial infarction. They showed that infusion of AM significantly reduced myocardial infarct size, left ventricular end-diastolic pressure, and myocardial apoptotic death with concomitant Akt phosphorylation. However, pretreatment with wortmannin (a phosphatidylinositol 3-kinase [PI3K] inhibitor) abolished the beneficial effect of AM. Infusion of AM significantly attenuated the myocardial ischemia/reperfusion injury. They concluded that cardioprotective effects of AM on ischemia/reperfusion injury might be mainly due to antiapoptotic effects of AM via a PI3K/Akt-dependent pathway. Thus, AM may have an anti-remodeling effect in acute myocardial infarction.

(4) Pulmonary Hypertension

AM has antiproliferative effects in vascular smooth muscle cells and cardiac fibroblasts and AM also inhibits vascular smooth muscle cell migration and hypertrophy in cultured neonatal cardiac myocytes. Yoshihara et al. (Yoshihara et al., 1998) reported the beneficial effect of long-term AM infusion in pulmonary hypertension and right ventricular hypertrophy induced by the administration of monocrotaline. Chronic infusion of AM significantly lessened the increase in right ventricular systolic pressure and the ratio of right ventricular weight. AM also attenuated the medial thickening of the pulmonary artery. These results suggest that chronic infusion of AM attenuates the pulmonary hypertension and right ventricular hypertrophy in rats treated with monocrotaline at least in part via an inhibitory effect on pulmonary arterial remodeling. These findings are consistent with recent studies which showed that chronic inhalation of AM inhibited the development of pulmonary hypertension (Nagaya et al., 2003).

These findings support the concept of AM as a protective peptide in cardiovascular disease and suggest that AM administration may be a new therapeutic approach.

REFERENCES

Ebara T, Miura K, Okumura M, Matsuura T, Kim S, Yukimura T, Iwao H. (1994) Effect of adrenomedullin on renal hemodynamics and functions in dogs. Eur J Pharmacol. 263:69-73.

Hirata Y, Hayakawa H, Suzuki Y, Suzuki E, Ikenouchi H, Kohmoto O, Kimura K, Kitamura K, Eto T, Kangawa K, Matsuo H, Omata M (1995) Mechanisms of adrenomedullin-inducedvasodilation in the rat kidney. Hypertension 25:790-795

Ishiyama Y, Kitamura K, Ichiki Y, Nakamura S, Kida O, Kangawa K, Eto T

(1993) Hemodynamic effects of a novel hypotensive peptide, human adrenomedullin, in rats. Eur J Pharmacol 241:271-273

Gardiner SM, Kemp PA, March JE, Bennett T (1995) Regional haemodynamic effects of human and rat adrenomedullin in conscious rats. Br J Pharmacol 114:584-591

Khan AI, Kato J, Kitamura K, Kangawa K, Eto T. (1997) Hypotensive effect of chronically infused adrenomedullin in conscious Wistar-Kyoto and spontaneously hypertensive rats. Clin Exp Pharmacol Physiol. 24:139-42.

Khan AI, Kato J, Ishiyama Y, Kitamura K, Kangawa K, Eto T. (1997) Effect of chronically infused adrenomedullin in two-kidney, one-clip hypertensive rats. Eur J Pharmacol. 333:187-90.

Kitamura K, Kangawa K, Kawamoto M, Ichiki Y, Nakamura S, Matsuo H, Eto T. (1993) Adrenomedullin: a novel hypotensive peptide isolated from human pheochromocytoma. Biochem Biophys Res Commun. 192:553-60.

Lainchbury JG, Nicholls MG, Espiner EA, Yandle TG, Lewis LK, Richards AM. (1999) Bioactivity and interactions of adrenomedullin and brain natriuretic peptide in patients with heart failure. Hypertension. 34:70-5.

McGregor DO, Troughton RW, Frampton C, Lynn KL, Yandle T, Richards AM, Nicholls MG. (2001) Hypotensive and natriuretic actions of adrenomedullin in subjects with chronic renal impairment. Hypertension. 37:1279-84.

Miura K, Ebara T, Okumura M, Matsuura T, Kim S, Yukimura T, Iwao H (1995) Attenuation of adrenomedullin-induced renal vasodilatation by NG-nitro L-arginine but not glibenclamide. Br J Pharmacol 115:917-924

Mori Y, Nishikimi T, Kobayashi N, Ono H, Kangawa K, Matsuoka H. (2002) Long-term adrenomedullin infusion improves survival in malignant hypertensive rats. Hypertension. 40: 107-13.

Nagaya N, Nishikimi T, Uematsu M, Nagaya N, Nishikimi T, Horio T, Yoshihara F, Kanazawa A, Matsuo H, Kangawa K. (1999) Cardiovascular and renal effects of adrenomedullin in rats with heart failure. Am J Physiol. 276:R213-8.

Nagaya N, Nishikimi T, Uematsu M, Satoh T, Oya H, Kyotani S, Sakamaki F, Ueno K, Nakanishi N, Miyatake K, Kangawa K. (2000a) Haemodynamic and hormonal effects of adrenomedullin in patients with pulmonary hypertension. Heart. 84:653-8.

Nagaya N, Satoh T, Nishikimi T, Uematsu M, Furuichi S, Sakamaki F, Oya H, Kyotani S, Nakanishi N, Goto Y, Masuda Y, Miyatake K, Kangawa K. (2000b) Hemodynamic, renal, and hormonal effects of adrenomedullin infusion in patients with congestive heart failure. Circulation. 101:498-503.

Nagaya N, Okumura H, Uematsu M, Shimizu W, Ono F, Shirai M, Mori H, Miyatake K, Kangawa K. (2003) Repeated inhalation of adrenomedullin ameliorates pulmonary hypertension and survival in monocrotaline rats. Am J Physiol Heart Circ Physiol. 285:H2125-31.

Nakamura M, Yoshida H, Makita S, Arakawa N, Niinuma H, Hiramori K (1997) Potent and long-lasting vasodilatory effects of adrenomedullin in humans. Comparisons between normal subjects and patients with chronic heart failure. Circulation 95:1214-1221

Nishikimi T, Yoshihara F, Kanazawa A, Okano I, Horio T, Nagaya N, Yutani C, Matsuo H, Matsuoka H, Kangawa K. (2001) Role of increased circulating and renal adrenomedullin in rats with malignant hypertension. Am J Physiol Regul Integr Comp Physiol. 281:R2079-87.

Nishikimi T, Mori Y, Kobayashi N, Tadokoro K, Wang X, Akimoto K, Yoshihara F, Kangawa K, Matsuoka H. (2002) Renoprotective effect of chronic adrenomedullin infusion in Dahl salt-sensitive rats. Hypertension. 39:1077-82.

Nishikimi T, Yoshihara F, Horinaka S, Kobayashi N, Mori Y, Tadokoro K,

Akimoto K, Minamino N, Kangawa K, Matsuoka H. (2003) Chronic administration of adrenomedullin attenuates transition from left ventricular hypertrophy to heart failure in rats. Hypertension. 42:1034-41.

Okumura H, Nagaya N, Itoh T, Okano I, Hino J, Mori K, Tsukamoto Y, Ishibashi-Ueda H, Miwa S, Tambara K, Toyokuni S, Yutani C, Kangawa K. (2004) Adrenomedullin infusion attenuates myocardial ischemia/reperfusion injury through the hosphatidylinositol 3-kinase/Akt-dependent pathway. Circulation. 109:242-8.

Rademaker MT, Charles CJ, Lewis LK, Yandle TG, Cooper GJ, Coy DH, Richards AM, Nicholls MG. (1997) Beneficial hemodynamic and renal effects of adrenomedullin in an ovine model of heart failure. Circulation. 96:1983-90.

Rademaker MT, Charles CJ, Cooper GJ, Coy DH, Espiner EA, Lewis LK, Nicholls MG, Richards AM. (2002a) Combined endopeptidase inhibition and adrenomedullin in sheep with experimental heart failure. Hypertension. 39:93-8.

Rademaker MT, Charles CJ, Espiner EA, Nicholls MG, Richards AM. (2002b) Long-term adrenomedullin administration in experimental heart failure. Hypertension. 40:667-72.

Parkes DG, May CN (1997) Direct cardiac and vascular actions of adrenomedullin in conscious sheep. Br J Pharmacol 120:1179-1185

Troughton RW, Lewis LK, Yandle TG, Richards AM, Nicholls MG.(2000) Hemodynamic, hormone, and urinary effects of adrenomedullin infusion in essential hypertension. Hypertension. 36:588-93.

Yoshihara F, Nishikimi T, Horio T, Yutani C, Takishita S, Matsuo H, Ohe T, Kangawa K. (1998) Chronic infusion of adrenomedullin reduces pulmonary hypertension and lessens right ventricular hypertrophy in rats administered monocrotaline. Eur J Pharmacol. 355:33-9.

12

THERAPEUTIC POTENTIALS OF ADRENOMEDULLIN FOR HEART FAILURE AND PULMONARY HYPERTENSION

Noritoshi Nagaya[1], Toshio Nishikimi[2], and Kenji Kangawa[3]

[1]*Department of Regenerative Medicine and Tissue Engineering, National Cardiovascular Center Research Institute, Osaka, Japan,* [2]*Department of Hypertension and Cardiorenal Medicine, Dokkyo University School of Medicine, Mibu, Tochigi, Japan, and* [3] *Department of Biochemistry, National Cardiovascular Center Research Institute, Osaka, Japan.*

INTRODUCTION

Earlier studies have shown that plasma adrenomedullin (AM) level is increased in patients with heart failure (Nishikimi et al., 1995) or pulmonary hypertension (Kakishita et al., 1999). Plasma AM level is increased in proportion to the severity of these diseases. Tissue levels of AM peptide and mRNA have also been shown to be increased in heart, kidney and lungs in rats with heart failure (Nishikimi et al., 1997). Taking together its potent vasodilatory, renal, and endocrine effect (see chapter 5 in detail), AM may be involved in the regulation of the body fluid and vascular tone in cardiovascular disease. In addition, AM has a variety of biological effects which are necessary for the treatment of congestive heart failure and pulmonary hypertension. This review summarizes the therapeutic potential of AM for the treatment of heart failure and pulmonary hypertension.

1. AM THERAPY IN HEART FAILURE

Experimental studies have shown that infusion of AM causes vasodilatation, diuresis and natriuresis in normal animals (Majid et al., 1996; Parkes et al., 1997). AM also increases cardiac output and left ventricular contractility in vivo (Parkes et al., 1997) and exerts a direct inotropic effect in vitro (Szokodi et al., 1998). These findings suggest that AM may have beneficial hemodynamic effects in heart failure. Thus, we investigated the therapeutic potential of AM infusion for the treatment of heart failure in humans.

(1) Vasodilatation

The vasodilatory effect is mediated by cAMP-dependent (Ishizaka et al., 1994) and nitric oxide-dependent mechanisms (Nakamura et al., 1997). Intravenous infusion of AM significantly decreased mean arterial pressure in patients with congestive heart failure (Fig. 1) (Nagaya et al., 2000a). The increase in cAMP in smooth muscle cells by AM activates protein kinase A, resulting in the decrease in calcium content in smooth muscle cells. It is therefore possible that AM may relax vascular smooth muscle through a cAMP/protein kinase A-dependent mechanism. The fall in mean arterial pressure was associated with a significant increase in heart rate (Nagaya et al., 2000a). Infusion of AM caused a greater and more prolonged reduction of mean arterial pressure than that of an equimolar amount of atrial natriuretic peptide (ANP) (Oya et al., 2000), which is already used as a therapeutic agent in heart failure. Unlike the marked effects of AM on arterial pressure, the reduction in pulmonary capillary wedge pressure (PCWP) by AM was smaller than that by ANP. AM may play an important role in the regulation of cardiac afterload but not in that of cardiac preload. Interestingly, AM significantly decreased mean pulmonary arterial pressure and pulmonary vascular resistance in patients with congestive heart failure. It has been reported that there are many binding sites for AM in the lung (Owji et al., 1995), and that AM preferentially dilates pulmonary arterial resistance vessels (Lippton et al., 1994). Circulating AM has been shown to be increased and to be partially metabolized in the lungs of patients with pulmonary hypertension (Yoshibayashi et al., 1997). These findings raise the possibility that AM plays a role in regulation of pulmonary vascular tone in patients with heart failure.

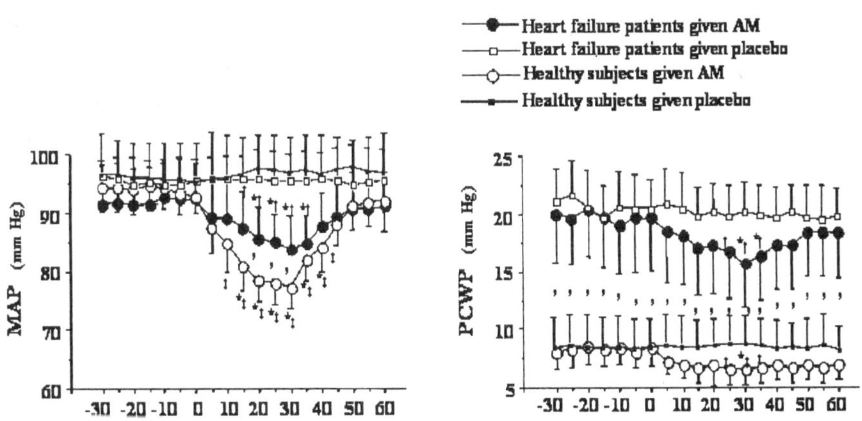

Figure 1. Changes in mean arterial pressure (MAP) and pulmonary capillary wedge pressure (PCWP) during infusion of AM or placebo. Data are mean ± SEM. *P < 0.05 vs value at time 0; †P < 0.05 vs heart failure patients given placebo; P < 0.05 vs healthy subjects given placebo; §P < 0.05, heart failure patients given AM vs healthy subjects given AM.

(2) Inotropic Effect

We have demonstrated that infusion of AM markedly increased cardiac index and stroke volume index in patients with congestive heart failure (Fig. 2) (Nagaya et al., 2000a). This is consistent with results obtained from a previous animal study using conscious sheep (Parkes et al., 1997).

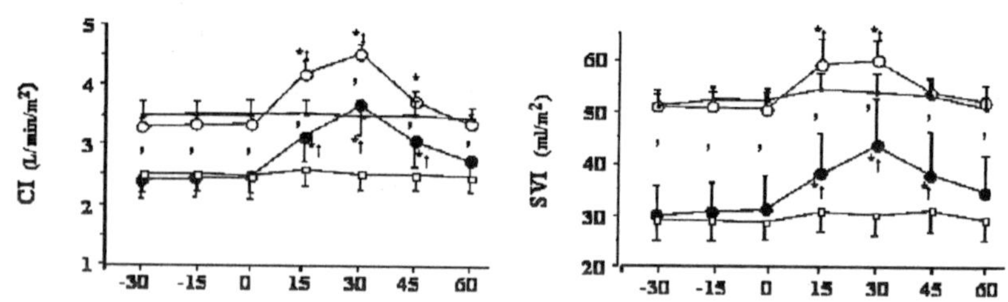

Figure 2. Changes in cardiac index (CI) and stroke volume index (SVI) during infusion of AM or placebo. Data are mean ± SEM. *$P < 0.05$ vs value at time 0; †$P < 0.05$ vs heart failure patients given placebo; $P < 0.05$ vs healthy subjects given placebo; §$P < 0.05$, heart failure patients given AM vs healthy subjects given AM.

Considering the strong vasodilator effect of AM, a significant decrease in mean arterial pressure may be responsible for increased cardiac index during infusion. On the other hand, a recent binding study has shown abundant binding sites for AM in the ventricular myocardium (Owji et al., 1995). In fact, AM has been shown to increase cardiac cAMP, which is known to mediate the positive inotropic action of ß-adrenergic stimulants. Alternatively, Szokodi et al have shown that AM produces a positive inotropic action through cAMP-independent mechanisms (Szokodi et al., 1998). AM caused greater increases in cardiac index and stroke volume index than ANP which has no direct effect on contractility (Oya H et al., 2000). These findings suggest that the increase in cardiac index by AM may be attributable not only to the fall in cardiac afterload but also to the direct positive inotropic action of AM.

(3) Diuretic and Natriuretic Effects

Systemically administered AM slightly, but significantly increased urine volume and urinary sodium excretion in patients with congestive heart failure, consistent with the results obtained from earlier animal studies (Majid et al., 1996; Rademaker et al., 1997). However, AM did not significantly increase creatinine clearance. Edwards et al have reported that AM dose-dependently increases intracellular cAMP levels in the cortical thick ascending limb and distal convoluted tubule dissected from rat kidney (Edwards et al., 1996). These findings suggest that AM can directly inhibit tubular sodium reabsorption. However, renal responses to AM were smaller than those to ANP which increases renal blood flow and glomerular filtration rate in a dose-dependent manner (Brenner et al., 1990). Because renal effects of systemically administered AM are relatively weak, significance of AM in the treatment of renal dysfunction remains to be determined.

(4) Inhibition of Aldosterone Production

The renin-angiotensin-aldosterone system is known to be excessively activated in patients with heart failure, leading to adverse effects. Interestingly, infusion of AM significantly decreased plasma aldosterone in patients with congestive heart failure, although there was no significant change in plasma rennin (Nagaya et al., 2000a). In vitro, AM has been shown to inhibit Ang II-induced secretion of aldosterone from dispersed rat adrenal zona glomerulosa cells (Yamaguchi et al., 1995). Thus, it is interesting to speculate that AM may play a compensatory role in the pathophysiology of heart failure by inhibiting the augmented production of aldosterone.

(5) Various Cardioprotective Effects

AM has been shown to be a possible endogenous suppressor of myocyte hypertrophy and fibroblast proliferation (Tsuruda et al., 1998; Tsuruda et al., 1999). In vitro studies have shown that AM inhibits the migration and proliferation of vascular smooth muscle cells (Horio et al., 1995; Kano et al., 1996). AM has anti-apoptotic effects on cardiomyocytes via phospatidylinositol 3-kinase (PI3K)/Akt pathway (Okumura et al., 2004). In addition, AM has been shown to inhibit vascular endothelial cell apoptosis (Kim et al., 2002) and induce angiogenesis through the activation of PI3K/Akt pathway (Tokunaga et al., 2004). Thus, AM has protective effects on myocardium and vasculature, which may have beneficial effects in patients with congestive heart failure.

2. AM THEREAPY IN PULMONARY HYPERTENSION

Primary pulmonary hypertension (PPH) is a rare but life-threatening disease characterized by progressive pulmonary hypertension, ultimately producing right ventricular failure and death (Rich et al., 1987). Median survival is considered to be 2.8 years from the time of diagnosis. Because the presence of endothelial injury in the pulmonary vascular bed develops pulmonary vasoconstriction, smooth muscle cell proliferation, and in situ thrombosis (Archer et al., 2000), a variety of vasodilators, anti-proliferative agents, and anticoagulants have been proposed as therapeutic agents of PPH. Despite therapeutic medical advances including prostacyclin therapy (Barst et al., 1996; McLaughlin et al., 1998), some patients ultimately require heart-lung or lung transplantation (Pasque et al., 1991). Therefore, a novel therapeutic strategy is desirable for the treatment of pulmonary hypertension including PPH. Experimental studies have shown that AM plays an important role in the regulation of pulmonary vascular tone and vascular remodeling. Thus, we investigated the therapeutic potential of AM administration for the treatment of pulmonary hypertension in humans. This review will summarize the effects of two types of AM delivery systems: intravenous administration and inhalation of AM peptide.

(1) Intravenous Administration

Intralobar arterial infusion of AM causes dose-related decreases in pulmonary vascular resistance under conditions of high pulmonary vascular tone (Heaton et al. 1995; Lippton et al., 1994). The vasodilatory effect is mediated by cAMP-dependent and nitric oxide-dependent mechanisms. Thus, AM is known to be one of the most potent endogenous vasodilators in the pulmonary vascular bed. However, little information is available regarding the hemodynamic effects of intravenously administered AM in patients with pulmonary hypertension. Accordingly, we examined the hemodynamic and hormonal responses to intravenous infusion of AM (0.05 μg/kg/min) or placebo were examined in 13 patients with pulmonary arterial hypertension including PPH (Nagaya et al. 2000b). Because AM-induced hypotension may cause adverse effects in patients with pulmonary hypertension, we used a relatively low dose of AM. Intravenous infusion of AM increased plasma AM level in patients with pulmonary hypertension (15 ± 1 to 48 ± 8 fmol/ml). Infusion of AM significantly decreased pulmonary vascular resistance by 32% without inducing a marked hypotension. The hemodynamic effects of AM lasted at least 15 min after the end of infusion. These results suggest that AM has potent, relatively long-lasting pulmonary vasodilator activities in patients with pulmonary hypertension. We have shown that administered AM increases plasma cAMP, but not cGMP, in patients with pulmonary hypertension, in association with its hemodynamic effects. The increase in cAMP in smooth muscle cells by AM activates protein kinase A, resulting in the decrease in calcium content in smooth muscle cells. It is therefore possible that AM may relax vascular smooth muscle through a cAMP/protein kinase A-dependent mechanism. On the other hand, Nossaman et al have shown that AM regulates pulmonary vascular tone in rats through an endothelium-derived nitric oxide-dependent mechanism (Nossaman et al. 1996). Because the vascular effects of AM are known to vary with species and vascular regions, further studies are necessary to elucidate the mechanisms responsible for pulmonary vasodilator activity of AM in humans.

Intravenous infusion of AM markedly increased cardiac index in patients with pulmonary hypertension (Nagaya et al. 2000b), consistent with our previous results from left sided heart failure. Considering the strong vasodilator activity of AM in the systemic and pulmonary vasculature, the significant decrease in cardiac afterload may be responsible for increased cardiac index with AM. On the other hand, AM produces a positive inotropic action through cAMP-independent mechanisms. These findings suggest that the increase in cardiac index may be attributable not only to a fall in cardiac afterload but also to the direct positive inotropic action of AM.

It appears that a number of similarities in pharmacological actions, i.e. vasodilatation, cardiac effect, and cAMP production, exist between AM and prostacyclin that is used for reducing pulmonary resistance in PPH. Unlike prostacyclin, however, AM has diuretic and natriuretic activities. AM inhibits inflammation and aldosterone production (Clementi et al., 1999; Yamaguchi et al. 1995). Thus, these biological effects may be the advantages of AM over prostacyclin in respect of therapeutic effectiveness. Exogenously administered AM at a pharmacological level increased plasma cAMP in association with hemodynamic effects. Thus, additional administration of AM may be effective in patients with pulmonary hypertension.

(2) Inhalation Therapy

The goal of vasodilator therapy for patients with PPH is to reduce pulmonary vascular resistance without producing systemic hypotension, and improve quality of life and survival. We have shown that intravenous administration of AM markedly decreases pulmonary vascular resistance in patients with pulmonary hypertension (Nagaya et al. 2000b). Nevertheless, systemically administered AM decreases systemic arterial pressure, which may be harmful in treating patients with PPH. Recently, inhalation of aerosolized prostacyclin and its analogue, iloprost, has been shown to cause pulmonary vasodilation without systemic hypotension in patients with PPH (Hoeper et al.

2000). In addition, inhalant application of vasodilators does not impair gas exchange because the ventilation-matched deposition of drug in the alveoli causes pulmonary vasodilation matched to ventilated areas. In clinical settings, inhalation therapy may be more simple, noninvasive, and comfortable than continuous intravenous infusion therapy. Thus, the purpose of this study was to investigate the effects of AM inhalation on hemodynamics and exercise capacity in patients with PPH.

Interestingly, Champion et al have shown that intratracheal gene transfer of calcitonin gene-related peptide (CGRP), a member of the same peptide family as AM, to bronchial epithelial cells attenuates chronic hypoxia-induced pulmonary hypertension in the mouse (Champion et al., 2000). These results raise the possibility that intratracheal delivery of a vasodilator peptide may be sufficient to alter pulmonary vascular function. In fact, inhalation of AM significantly decreased pulmonary vascular resistance in patients with pulmonary hypertension, whereas it did not alter systemic arterial pressure or systemic vascular resistance (Nagaya et al., 2004). The ratio of pulmonary vascular resistance to systemic vascular resistance was significantly reduced by AM inhalation. These results suggest that inhaled AM improves hemodynamics with pulmonary selectivity. This is consistent with earlier findings that inhaled prostacyclin or its analogue, iloprost, acts transepithelially with pulmonary selectivity and improves pulmonary hypertension.

We examined the long-term effects of inhaled AM in monocrotaline (MCT)-induced pulmonary hypertension rats (Nagaya et al., 2003). AM or saline was inhaled as an aerosol using an ultrasonic nebulizer, for 30 min, 4 times a day. Repeated inhalation of AM for three weeks markedly decreased mean pulmonary arterial pressure and pulmonary vascular resistance in MCT rats without systemic hypotension. The potent, long-lasting pulmonary vasodilator effect of inhaled AM may contribute to the strong inhibition of the development of pulmonary hypertension. In addition, considering intermittent delivery of AM to the lungs, the chronic effects of inhaled AM appear to go beyond acute pulmonary vasodilation. Inhalation of AM inhibited an increase in the medial wall thickness of peripheral pulmonary arteries of MCT rats. In vitro studies have shown that AM inhibits the migration and proliferation of vascular smooth muscle cells (Horio et al., 1995; Kano et al., 1996). Given the known potent vasoprotective effects of AM such as vasodilation and inhibition of smooth muscle cell migration and proliferation, it is interesting to speculate that AM trapped in the bronchial epithelium or alveoli leaks to the pulmonary arteries to maintain pulmonary vascular integrity in MCT rats. Importantly, Kaplan-Meier analysis demonstrated that the 6-week survival rate for MCT rats treated with aerosolized AM was significantly high (70%) as compared with 10% in those given saline (Nagaya et al., 2003). Thus, treatment with aerosolized AM may be an alternative approach for severe pulmonary hypertension that is refractory to conventional therapy. Although further studies are necessary to maximize the efficiency and reproducibility of pulmonary AM delivery, combining AM inhalation therapy with other modalities that have a different mode of action may have beneficial effects in patients with PPH.

SUMMARY

This article described the therapeutic potential of AM for the treatment of congestive heart failure and pulmonary hypertension. Baseline plasma AM is significantly higher in patients with these diseases. Nevertheless, exogenously administered AM at a pharmacological level induces hemodynamic improvement. These beneficial effects of AM are mediated by vasodilation, positive isotropic effects, diuresis, natriuresis, inhibition of aldosterone, and et al. Thus, AM supplementation may be a new therapeutic strategy for the treatment of congestive heart failure and pulmonary hypertension. Further studies are necessary to examine whether long-term administration of AM improves survival in such patients.

REFERENCES

Archer S, and Rich S. (2000) Primary pulmonary hypertension: a vascular biology and transnational research "Work in progress". Circulation 102:2781-2791.

Barest RJ, Rubin LJ, Long WA, McGoon MD, Rich S, Badesch DB, Groves BM, Tapson VF, Bourge RC, and Brundage BH, et al. (1996) A comparison of continuous intravenous epoprostenol (prostacyclin) with conventional therapy for primary pulmonary hypertension. N Engl J Med 334:296-302.

Brenner BM, Ballermann BJ, Gunning ME, and Zeidel ML. (1990) Diverse biological actions of natriuretic peptide. Physiol Rev 70:665-699.

Champion HC, Bivalacqua TJ, Toyoda K, Heistad DD, Hyman AL, and Kadowitz PJ. (2000) In vivo gene transfer of prepro-calcitonin gene-related peptide to the lung attenuates chronic hypoxia-induced pulmonary hypertension in the mouse. Circulation 101:923-930.

Clementi G, Caruso A, Cutuli VM, Prato A, Mangano NG, and Amico-Roxas M. (1999) Antiinflammatory activity of adrenomedullin in the acetic acid peritonitis in rats. Life Sci 65:PL203-208.

Edwards RM, Trizna W, Stack E, and Aiyar N. (1996) Effect of adrenomedullin on cAMP levels along the rat nephron: comparison with CGRP. Am J Physiol 271:F895-F899.

Heaton J, Lin B, Chang JK, Steinberg S, Hyman A, and Lippton H. (1995) Pulmonary vasodilation to adrenomedullin: a novel peptide in humans. Am J Physiol 268:H2211-2215.

Hoeper MM, Schwarze M, Ehlerding S, Adler-Schuermeyer A, Spiekerkoetter E, Niedermeyer J, Hamm M, and Fabel H. (2000) Long-term treatment of primary pulmonary hypertension with aerosolized iloprost, a prostacyclin analogue. N Engl J Med 342:1866-1870.

Horio T, Kohno M, Kano H, Ikeda M, Yasunari K, Yokokawa K, Minami M, and Takeda T. (1995) Adrenomedullin as a novel antimigration factor of vascular smooth muscle cells. Circ Res 77:660-664.

Kakishita M, Nishikimi T, Okano Y, Satoh T, Kyotani S, Nagaya N, Fukushima K, Nakanishi N, Takishita S, Miyata A, Kangawa K, Matsuo H, and Kunieda T. (1999) Increased plasma levels of adrenomedullin in patients with pulmonary hypertension. Clin Sci (Lond) 96:33-39.

Kano H, Kohno M, Yasunari K, Yokokawa K, Horio T, Ikeda M, Minami M, Hanehira T, Takeda T, and Yoshikawa J. (1996) Adrenomedullin as a novel antiproliferative factor of vascular smooth muscle cells. J Hypertens 14:209-213.

Kim W, Moon SO, Sung MJ, Kim SH, Lee S, Kim HJ, Koh GY, and Park SK. (2002) Protective effect of adrenomedullin in mannitol-induced apoptosis. Apoptosis 7:527-535.

Lippton H, Chang J-K, Hao Q, Summer W, and Hyman AL. (1994) Adrenomedullin dilates the pulmonary vascular bed in vivo. J Appl Physiol 76:2154-2156.

Majid DS, Kadowitz PJ, Coy DH, Navar LG. (1996) Renal responses to intra-arterial administration of adrenomedullin in dogs. Am J Physiol. 1996;270:F200-205.

McLaughlin VV, Genthner DE, Panella MM, and Rich S. (1998) Reduction in pulmonary vascular resistance with long-term epoprostenol (prostacyclin) therapy in primary pulmonary hypertension. N Engl J Med 338:273-277.

Nagaya N, Kyotani S, Uematsu M, Ueno K, Oya H, Nakanishi N, Shirai M, Mori H, Miyatake K, and Kangawa K. (2004) Effects of adrenomedullin inhalation on hemodynamics and exercise capacity in patients with idiopathic pulmonary arterial hypertension. Circulation 109:351-356.

Nagaya N, Okumura H, Uematsu M, Shimizu W, Ono F, Shirai M, Mori H, Miyatake K, and Kangawa K. (2003) Repeated inhalation of adrenomedullin ameliorates pulmonary hypertension and survival in monocrotaline rats. Am J Physiol Heart Circ Physiol 285:H2125-2131.

Nagaya N, Satoh T, Nishikimi T, Uematsu M, Furuichi S, Sakamaki F, Oya H, Kyotani S, Nakanishi N, Goto Y, Masuda Y, Miyatake K, and Kangawa K. (2000a) Hemodynamic, renal, and hormonal effects of adrenomedullin infusion in patients with congestive heart failure. Circulation 101:498-503.

Nagaya N, Nishikimi T, Uematsu M, Satoh T, Oya H, Kyotani S, Sakamaki F, Ueno K, Nakanishi N, Miyatake K, and Kangawa K. (2000b) Haemodynamic and hormonal effects of adrenomedullin in patients with pulmonary hypertension. Heart 84:653-658.

Nakamura M, Yoshida H, Makita S, Arakawa N, Niinuma H, and Hiramori K. (1997) Potent and long-lasting vasodilatory effects of adrenomedullin in humans: comparisons between normal subjects and patients with chronic heart failure. Circulation 95:1214-1221.

Nishikimi T, Saito Y, Kitamura K, Ishimitsu T, Eto T, Kangawa K, Matsuo H, Omae T, and Matsuoka H. (1995) Increased plasma levels of adrenomedullin in patients with heart failure. J Am Coll Cardiol 26:1424-1431.

Nishikimi T, Horio T, Sasaki T, Yoshihara F, Takishita S, Miyata A, Matsuo H, Kangawa K. (1997) Cardiac production and secretion of adrenomedullin are increased in heart failure. Hypertension. 30:1369-1375.

Nossaman BD, Feng CJ, Kaye AD, DeWitt B, Coy DH, Murphy WA, and Kadowitz PJ. (1996) Pulmonary vasodilator responses to adrenomedullin are reduced by NOS inhibitors in rats but not in cats. Am J Physiol 270:L782-789.

Okumura H, Nagaya N, Itoh T, Okano I, Hino J, Mori K, Tsukamoto Y, Ishibashi-Ueda H, Miwa S, Tambara K, Toyokuni S, Yutani C, and Kangawa K. (2004) Adrenomedullin infusion attenuates myocardial ischemia/reperfusion injury through the phosphatidylinositol 3-kinase/Akt-dependent pathway. Circulation 109:242-248.

Owji AA, Smith DM, Coppock HA, Morgan DG, Bhogal R, Ghatei MA, and Bloom SR. (1995) An abundant and specific binding site for the novel vasodilator adrenomedullin in the rat. Endocrinology 136:2127-2134.

Oya H, Nagaya N, Furuichi S, Nishikimi T, Ueno K, Nakanishi N, Yamagishi M, Kangawa K, and Miyatake K. (2000) Comparison of intravenous adrenomedullin with atrial natriuretic peptide in patients with congestive heart failure. Am J Cardiol. 86:94-98.

Parkes DG, and May CN. (1997) Direct cardiac and vascular actions of adrenomedullin in conscious sheep. Br J Pharmacol 120:1179-1185.

Pasque MK, Trulock EP, Kaiser LR, and Cooper JD. (1991) Single lung transplantation for pulmonary hypertension: three month hemodynamic follow-up. Circulation 84:2275-2279.

Rademaker MT, Charles CJ, Lewis LK, Yandle TG, Cooper GJ, Coy DH, Richards AM, and Nicholls MG. (1997) Beneficial hemodynamic and renal effects of adrenomedullin in an ovine model of heart failure. Circulation 96:1983-1990.

Rich S, Dantzker DR, Ayres SM, Bergofsky EH, Brundage BH, Detre KM, Fishman AP, Goldring RM, Groves BM, and Koerner SK. (1987) Primary pulmonary hypertension: a national prospective study. Ann Intern Med 107:216-223.

Szokodi I, Kinnunen P, Tavi P, Weckstrom M, Toth M, and Ruskoaho H. (1998) Evidence for cAMP-independent mechanisms mediating the effects of adrenomedullin, a new inotropic peptide. Circulation 97:1062-1070.

Tokunaga N, Nagaya N, Shirai M, Tanaka E, Ishibashi-Ueda H, Harada-Shiba M, Kanda M, Ito T, Shimizu W, Tabata Y, Uematsu M, Nishigami K, Sano S, Kangawa K, and Mori H. (2004) Adrenomedullin gene transfer induces therapeutic angiogenesis in a rabbit model of chronic hindlimb ischemia: benefits of a novel nonviral vector, gelatin. Circulation 109:526-531.

Tsuruda T, Kato J, Kitamura K, Kawamoto M, Kuwasako K, Imamura T, Koiwaya Y, Tsuji T, Kangawa K, and Eto T. (1999) An autocrine or a paracrine role of adrenomedullin in modulating cardiac fibroblast growth. Cardiovasc Res. 43:958-967.

Tsuruda T, Kato J, Kitamura K, Kuwasako K, Imamura T, Koiwaya Y, Tsuji T, Kangawa K, and Eto T. (1998) Adrenomedullin: a possible autocrine or paracrine inhibitor of hypertrophy of cardiomyocytes. Hypertension 31:505-510.

Yamaguchi T, Baba K, Doi Y, and Yano K. (1995) Effect of adrenomedullin on aldosterone secretion by dispersed rat adrenal zona glomerulosa cells. Life Sci 56:379-387.

Yoshibayashi M, Kamiya T, Kitamura K, Saito Y, Kangawa K, Nishikimi T, Matsuoka H, Eto T, and Matsuo H. (1997) Plasma levels of adrenomedullin in primary and secondary pulmonary hypertension in patients < 20 years of age. Am J Cardiol 79:1556-1558.

Index